Navane® (thiothixene) Capsules
(thiothixene hydrochloride) Concentrate

S0-DQZ-787

PRESCRIBING INFORMATION

ACTIONS. Navane is a psychotropic agent of the thioxanthene series. Navane possesses certain chemical and pharmacological similarities to the piperazine phenothiazines and differences from the aliphatic group of phenothiazines.

INDICATIONS. Navane is effective in the management of manifestations of psychotic disorders. Navane has not been evaluated in the management of behavioral complications in patients with mental retardation.

CONTRAINDICATIONS. Navane is contraindicated in patients with circulatory collapse, comatose states, central nervous system depression due to any cause, and blood dyscrasias. Navane is contraindicated in individuals who have shown hypersensitivity to the drug. It is not known whether there is a cross sensitivity between the thioxanthenes and the phenothiazine derivatives, but this possibility should be considered.

WARNINGS. Usage in Pregnancy—Safe use of Navane during pregnancy has not been established. Therefore, this drug should be given to pregnant patients only when, in the judgment of the physician, the expected benefits from the treatment exceed the possible risks to mother and fetus. Animal reproduction studies and clinical experience to date have not demonstrated any teratogenic effects.

In the animal reproduction studies with Navane, there was some decrease in conception rate and litter size, and an increase in resorption rate in rats and rabbits. Similar findings have been reported with other psychotropic agents. After repeated oral administration of Navane (thiothixene) to rats (5 to 15 mg/kg/day), rabbits (3 to 50 mg/kg/day), and monkeys (1 to 3 mg/kg/day) before and during gestation, no teratogenic effects were seen.

Usage in Children—The use of Navane in children under 12 years of age is not recommended because safe conditions for its use have not been established.

As is true with many CNS drugs, Navane may impair the mental and/or physical abilities required for the performance of potentially hazardous tasks such as driving a car or operating machinery, especially during the first few days of therapy. Therefore, the patient should be cautioned accordingly.

As in the case of other CNS-acting drugs, patients receiving Navane should be cautioned about the possible additive effects (which may include hypotension) with CNS depressants and with alcohol.

PRECAUTIONS. An antiemetic effect was observed in animal studies with Navane; since this effect may also occur in man, it is possible that Navane may mask signs of overdosage of toxic drugs and may obscure conditions such as intestinal obstruction and brain tumor.

In consideration of the known capability of Navane and certain other psychotropic drugs to precipitate convulsions, extreme caution should be used in patients with a history of convulsive disorders or those in a state of alcohol withdrawal, since it may lower the convulsive threshold. Although Navane potentiates the actions of the barbiturates, the dosage of the anticonvulsant therapy should not be reduced when Navane is administered concurrently.

Though exhibiting rather weak anticholinergic properties, Navane should be used with caution in patients who might be exposed to extreme heat or who are receiving atropine or related drugs.

Use with caution in patients with cardiovascular disease.

Caution as well as careful adjustment of the dosages is indicated when Navane (thiothixene) is used in conjunction with other CNS depressants.

Also, careful observation should be made for pigmentary retinopathy, and lenticular pigmentation (fine lenticular pigmentation has been noted in a small number of patients treated with Navane for prolonged periods). Blood dyscrasias (agranulocytosis, pancytopenia, thrombocytopenic purpura), and liver damage (jaundice, biliary stasis), have been reported with related drugs.

Neuroleptic drugs elevate prolactin levels; the elevation persists during chronic administration. Tissue culture experiments indicate that approximately one-third of human breast cancers are prolactin dependent *in vitro*, a factor of potential importance if the prescription of these drugs is contemplated in a patient with a previously detected breast cancer. Although disturbances such as galactorrhea, amenorrhea, gynecomastia, and impotence have been reported, the clinical significance of elevated serum prolactin levels is unknown for most patients. An increase in mammary neoplasms has been found in rodents after chronic administration of neuroleptic drugs. Neither clinical studies nor epidemiologic studies conducted to date, however, have shown an association between chronic administration of these drugs and mammary tumorigenesis; the available evidence is considered too limited to be conclusive at this time.

ADVERSE REACTIONS. NOTE: Not all of the following adverse reactions have been reported with Navane. However, since Navane has certain chemical and pharmacologic similarities to the phenothiazines, all of the known side effects and toxicity associated with phenothiazine therapy should be borne in mind when Navane is used.

Cardiovascular effects: Tachycardia, hypotension, lightheadedness, and syncope. In the event hypotension occurs, epinephrine should not be used as a pressor agent since a paradoxical further lowering of blood pressure may result. Nonspecific EKG changes have been observed in some patients receiving Navane (thiothixene). These changes are usually reversible and frequently disappear on continued Navane therapy. The incidence of these changes is lower than that observed with some phenothiazines. The clinical significance of these changes is not known.

CNS effects: Drowsiness, usually mild, may occur although it usually subsides with continuation of Navane therapy. The incidence of sedation appears similar to that of the piperazine group of phenothiazines but less than that of certain aliphatic phenothiazines. Restlessness, agitation and insomnia have been noted with Navane. Seizures and paradoxical exacerbation of psychotic symptoms have occurred with Navane infrequently.

Hyperreflexia has been reported in infants delivered from mothers having received structurally related drugs.

In addition, phenothiazine derivatives have been associated with cerebral edema and cerebrospinal fluid abnormalities.

Extrapyramidal symptoms, such as pseudo-parkinsonism, akathisia, and dystonia have been reported. Management of these extrapyramidal symptoms depends upon the type and severity. Rapid relief of acute symptoms may require the use of an injectable antiparkinson agent. More slowly emerging symptoms may be managed by reducing the dosage of Navane and/or administering an oral antiparkinson agent.

Persistent Tardive Dyskinesia: As with all antipsychotic agents tardive dyskinesia may appear in some patients on long term therapy or may occur after drug therapy has been discontinued. The risk seems to be greater in elderly patients on high-dose therapy, especially females. The symptoms are persistent and in some patients appear to be irreversible. The syndrome is characterized by rhythmical involuntary movements of the tongue, face, mouth or jaw (e.g., protrusion of tongue, puffing of cheeks, puckering of mouth, chewing movements). Sometimes these may be accompanied by involuntary movements of extremities.

There is no known effective treatment for tardive dyskinesia; antiparkinsonism agents usually do not alleviate the symptoms of this syndrome. It is suggested that all antipsychotic agents be discontinued if these symptoms appear.

Should it be necessary to reinstitute treatment, or increase the dosage of the agent, or switch to a different antipsychotic agent, the syndrome may be masked.

It has been reported that fine vermicular movements of the tongue may be an early sign of the syndrome and if the medication is stopped at that time, the syndrome may not develop.

Hepatic effects: Elevations of serum transaminase and alkaline phosphatase, usually transient, have been infrequently observed in some patients. No clinically confirmed cases of jaundice attributable to Navane (thiothixene) have been reported.

Hematologic effects: As is true with certain other psychotropic drugs, leukopenia and leucocytosis, which are usually transient, can occur occasionally with Navane. Other antipsychotic drugs have been associated with agranulocytosis, eosinophilia, hemolytic anemia, thrombocytopenia and pancytopenia.

Allergic reactions: Rash, pruritus, urticaria, photosensitivity and rare cases of anaphylaxis have been reported with Navane (thiothixene). Undue exposure to sunlight should be avoided. Although not experienced with Navane, exfoliative dermatitis and contact dermatitis (in nursing personnel), have been reported with certain phenothiazines.

Endocrine disorders: Lactation, moderate breast enlargement and amenorrhea have occurred in a small percentage of females receiving Navane. If persistent, this may necessitate a reduction in dosage or the discontinuation of therapy. Phenothiazines have been associated with false positive pregnancy tests, gynecomastia, hypoglycemia, hyperglycemia and glycosuria.

Autonomic effects: Dry mouth, blurred vision, nasal congestion, constipation, increased sweating, increased salivation and impotence have occurred infrequently with Navane therapy. Phenothiazines have been associated with miosis, mydriasis, and adynamic ileus.

Other adverse reactions: Hyperpyrexia, anorexia, nausea, vomiting, diarrhea, increase in appetite and weight, weakness or fatigue, polydipsia, and peripheral edema.

Although not reported with Navane, evidence indicates there is a relationship between phenothiazine therapy and the occurrence of a systemic lupus erythematosus-like syndrome.

NOTE: Sudden deaths have occasionally been reported in patients who have received certain phenothiazine derivatives. In some cases the cause of death was apparently cardiac arrest or asphyxia due to failure of the cough reflex. In others, the cause could not be determined nor could it be established that death was due to phenothiazine administration.

DOSAGE AND ADMINISTRATION. Dosage of Navane should be individually adjusted depending on the chronicity and severity of the condition. In general, small doses should be used initially and gradually increased to the optimal effective level, based on patient response.

Some patients have been successfully maintained on once-a-day Navane (thiothixene) therapy.

The use of Navane in children under 12 years of age is not recommended because safe conditions for its use have not been established.

In milder conditions, an initial dose of 2 mg three times daily. If indicated, a subsequent increase to 15 mg/day total daily dose is often effective.

In more severe conditions, an initial dose of 5 mg twice daily.

The usual optimal dose is 20 to 30 mg daily. If indicated, an increase to 60 mg/day total daily dose is often effective. Exceeding a total daily dose of 60 mg rarely increases the beneficial response.

OVERDOSAGE. Manifestations include muscular twitching, drowsiness and dizziness. Symptoms of gross overdosage may include CNS depression, rigidity, weakness, torticollis, tremor, salivation, dysphagia, hypotension, disturbances of gait, or coma.

Treatment: Essentially symptomatic and supportive. Early gastric lavage is helpful. Keep patient under careful observation and maintain an open airway, since involvement of the extrapyramidal system may produce dysphagia and respiratory difficulty in severe overdosage. If hypotension occurs, the standard measures for managing circulatory shock should be used (I.V. fluids and/or vasoconstrictors).

If a vasoconstrictor is needed, levarterenol and phenylephrine are the most suitable drugs. Other pressor agents, including epinephrine, are not recommended, since phenothiazine derivatives may reverse the usual pressor action of these agents and cause further lowering of blood pressure.

If CNS depression is present, recommended stimulants include amphetamine, dextroamphetamine, or caffeine and sodium benzoate. Stimulants that may cause convulsions (e.g., picrotoxin or pentylene-tetrazol) should be avoided. Extrapyramidal symptoms may be treated with antiparkinson drugs.

There are no data on the use of peritoneal or hemodialysis, but they are known to be of little value in phenothiazine intoxication.

HOW SUPPLIED. Navane (thiothixene) is available as capsules containing 1 mg, 2 mg, 5 mg, and 10 mg thiothixene in bottles of 100, 1,000, and unit-dose pack of 100 (10 x 10's). Navane is also available as capsules containing 20 mg of thiothixene in bottles of 100, 500, and unit-dose pack of 100 (10 x 10's).

Navane (thiothixene hydrochloride) Concentrate is available in 120 ml (4 oz.) bottles with an accompanying dropper calibrated at 2 mg, 3 mg, 4 mg, 5 mg, 6 mg, 8 mg, and 10 mg, and in 30 ml (1 oz.) bottles with an accompanying dropper calibrated at 2 mg, 3 mg, 4 mg, and 5 mg. Each ml contains thiothixene hydrochloride equivalent to 5 mg of thiothixene. Contains alcohol, U.S.P. 7.0% v/v. (small loss unavoidable).

Navane®
(thiothixene hydrochloride) Intramuscular For Injection/Intramuscular Solution

PRESCRIBING INFORMATION

ACTIONS. Navane is a psychotropic agent of the thioxanthene series. Navane possesses certain chemical and pharmacological similarities to the piperazine phenothiazines and differences from the aliphatic group of phenothiazines. Navane's mode of action has not been clearly established.

INDICATIONS. Navane is effective in the management of manifestations of psychotic disorders. Navane has not been evaluated in the management of behavioral complications in patients with mental retardation.

CONTRAINDICATIONS. Navane is contraindicated in patients with circulatory collapse, comatose states, central nervous system depression due to any cause, and blood dyscrasias. Navane is contraindicated in individuals who have shown hypersensitivity to the drug. It is not known whether there is a cross sensitivity between the thioxanthenes and the phenothiazine derivatives, but this possibility should be considered.

WARNINGS. Usage in Pregnancy—Safe use of Navane during pregnancy has not been established. Therefore, this drug should be given to pregnant patients only when, in the judgment of the physician, the expected benefits from the treatment exceed the possible risks to mother and fetus. Animal reproductive studies and clinical experience to date have not demonstrated any teratogenic effects.

In the animal reproduction studies with Navane, there was some decrease in conception rate and litter size, and an increase in resorption rate in rats and rabbits, changes which have been similarly reported with other psychotropic agents. After repeated oral administration of Navane (thiothixene hydrochloride) to rats (5 to 15 mg/kg/day), rabbits (3 to 50 mg/kg/day), and monkeys (1 to 3 mg/kg/day) before and during gestation, no teratogenic effects were seen. (See Precautions.)

Usage in Children—The use of Navane in children under 12 years of age is not recommended because safety and efficacy in the pediatric age group have not been established.

As is true with many CNS drugs, Navane may impair the mental and/or physical abilities required for the performance of potentially hazardous tasks such as driving a car or operating machinery, especially during the first few days of therapy. Therefore, the patient should be cautioned accordingly.

As in the case of other CNS-acting drugs, patients receiving Navane should be cautioned about the possible additive effects, (which may include hypotension) with CNS depressants and with alcohol.

PRECAUTIONS. An antiemetic effect was observed in animal studies with Navane; since this effect may also occur in man, it is possible that Navane may mask signs of overdosage of toxic drugs and may obscure conditions such as intestinal obstruction and brain tumor.

In consideration of the known capability of Navane and certain other psychotropic drugs to precipitate convulsions, extreme caution should be used in patients with a history of convulsive disorders, or those in a state of alcohol withdrawal since it may lower the convulsive threshold. Although Navane potentiates the actions of the barbiturates, the dosage of the anticonvulsant therapy should not be reduced when Navane is administered concurrently.

Caution as well as careful adjustment of the dosages is indicated when Navane is used in conjunction with other CNS depressants other than anticonvulsant drugs.

Though exhibiting rather weak anticholinergic properties, Navane (thiothixene hydrochloride) should be used with caution in patients who are known or suspected to have glaucoma, or who might be exposed to extreme heat, or who are receiving atropine or related drugs.

Use with caution in patients with cardiovascular disease.

Also, careful observation should be made for pigmentary retinopathy, and lenticular pigmentation (fine lenticular pigmentation has been noted in a small number of patients treated with Navane for prolonged periods). Blood dyscrasias (agranulocytosis, pancytopenia, thrombocytopenic purpura), and liver damage (jaundice, biliary stasis), have been reported with related drugs.

Undue exposure to sunlight should be avoided. Photosensitive reactions have been reported in patients on Navane.

As with all intramuscular preparations, Navane Intramuscular should be injected well within the body of a relatively large muscle. The preferred sites are the upper outer quadrant of the buttock (i.e., gluteus maximus) and the mid-lateral thigh.

The deltoid area should be used only if well developed such as in certain adults and older children, and then only with caution to avoid radial nerve injury. Intramuscular injections should not be made into the lower and mid-thirds of the upper arm. As with all intramuscular injections, aspiration is necessary to help avoid inadvertent injection into a blood vessel.

Neuroleptic drugs elevate prolactin levels; the elevation persists during chronic administration. Tissue culture experiments indicate that approximately one-third of human breast cancers are prolactin dependent *in vitro,* a factor of potential importance if the prescription of these drugs is contemplated in a patient with a previously detected breast cancer. Although disturbances such as galactorrhea, amenorrhea, gynecomastia, and impotence have been reported, the clinical significance of elevated serum prolactin levels is unknown for most patients. An increase in mammary neoplasms has been found in rodents after chronic administration of neuroleptic drugs. Neither clinical studies nor epidemiologic studies conducted to date, however, have shown an association between chronic administration of these drugs and mammary tumorigenesis; the available evidence is considered too limited to be conclusive at this time.

ADVERSE REACTIONS. NOTE: Not all of the following adverse reactions have been reported with Navane (thiothixene hydrochloride). However, since Navane has certain chemical and pharmacologic similarities to the phenothiazines, all of the known side effects and toxicity associated with phenothiazine therapy should be borne in mind when Navane is used.

Cardiovascular effects: Tachycardia, hypotension, lightheadedness, and syncope. In the event hypotension occurs, epinephrine should not be used as a pressor agent since a paradoxical further lowering of blood pressure may result. Nonspecific EKG changes have been observed in some patients receiving Navane. These changes are usually reversible and frequently disappear on continued Navane therapy. The clinical significance of these changes is not known.

CNS effects: Drowsiness, usually mild, may occur although it usually subsides with continuation of Navane therapy. The incidence of sedation appears similar to that of the piperazine group of phenothiazines, but less than that of certain aliphatic phenothiazines. Restlessness, agitation and insomnia have been noted with Navane. Seizures and paradoxical exacerbation of psychotic symptoms have occurred with Navane infrequently.

Hyperreflexia has been reported in infants delivered from mothers having received structurally related drugs.

In addition, phenothiazine derivatives have been associated with cerebral edema and cerebrospinal fluid abnormalities.

Extrapyramidal symptoms, such as pseudo-parkinsonism, akathisia, and dystonia have been reported. Management of these extrapyramidal symptoms depends upon the type and severity. Rapid relief of acute symptoms may require the use of an injectable antiparkinson agent. More slowly emerging symptoms may be managed by reducing the dosage of Navane (thiothixene hydrochloride) and/or administering an oral antiparkinson agent.

Persistent Tardive Dyskinesia: As with all antipsychotic agents tardive dyskinesia may appear in some patients on long term therapy or may occur after drug therapy has been discontinued. The risk seems to be greater in elderly patients on high-dose therapy, especially females. The symptoms are persistent and in some patients appear to be irreversible. The syndrome is characterized by rhythmical involuntary movements of the tongue, face, mouth or jaw (e.g., protrusion of tongue, puffing of cheeks, puckering of mouth, chewing movements). Sometimes these may be accompanied by involuntary movements of extremities.

There is no known effective treatment for tardive dyskinesia; antiparkinsonism agents usually do not alleviate the symptoms of this syndrome. It is suggested that all antipsychotic agents be discontinued if these symptoms appear.

Should it be necessary to reinstitute treatment, or increase the dosage of the agent, or switch to a different antipsychotic agent, the syndrome may be masked.

It has been reported that fine vermicular movements of the tongue may be an early sign of the syndrome and if the medication is stopped at that time, the syndrome may not develop.

Hepatic effects: Elevations of serum transaminase and alkaline phosphatase, usually transient, have been infrequently observed in some patients. No clinically confirmed cases of jaundice attributable to Navane (thiothixene hydrochloride) have been reported.

Hematologic effects: As is true with certain other psychotropic drugs, leukopenia and leucocytosis, which are usually transient, can occur occasionally with Navane. Other antipsychotic drugs have been associated with agranulocytosis, eosinophilia, hemolytic anemia, thrombocytopenia and pancytopenia.

Allergic reactions: Rash, pruritus, urticaria, and rare cases of anaphylaxis have been reported with Navane. Undue exposure to sunlight should be avoided. Although not experienced with Navane, exfoliative dermatitis, contact dermatitis (in nursing personnel), have been reported with certain phenothiazines.

Endocrine disorders: Lactation, moderate breast enlargement and amenorrhea have occurred in a small percentage of females receiving Navane. If persistent, this may necessitate a reduction in dosage or the discontinuation of therapy. Phenothiazines have been associated with false positive pregnancy tests, gynecomastia, hypoglycemia, hyperglycemia, and glycosuria.

Autonomic effects: Dry mouth, blurred vision, nasal congestion, constipation, increased sweating, increased salivation, and impotence have occurred infrequently with Navane (thiothixene hydrochloride) therapy. Phenothiazines have been associated with miosis, mydriasis, and adynamic ileus.

Other adverse reactions: Hyperpyrexia, anorexia, nausea, vomiting, diarrhea, increase in appetite and weight, weakness or fatigue, polydipsia and peripheral edema.

Although not reported with Navane, evidence indicates there is a relationship between phenothiazine therapy and the occurrence of a systemic lupus erythematosus-like syndrome.

NOTE: Sudden deaths have occasionally been reported in patients who have received certain phenothiazine derivatives. In some cases the cause of death was apparently cardiac arrest or asphyxia due to failure of the cough reflex. In others, the cause could not be determined nor could it be established that death was due to phenothiazine administration.

DOSAGE AND ADMINISTRATION. Preparation: Navane Intramuscular Solution is ready for use as supplied.

Navane Intramuscular For Injection must be reconstituted with 2.2 ml of Sterile Water for Injection.

For Intramuscular Use Only: Dosage of Navane should be individually adjusted depending on the chronicity and severity of the condition. In general, small doses should be used initially and gradually increased to the optimal effective level, based on patient response.

Usage in children under 12 years of age is not recommended.

Where more rapid control and treatment of acute behavior is desirable, the intramuscular form of Navane may be indicated. It is also of benefit where the very nature of the patient's symptomatology, whether acute or chronic, renders oral administration impractical or even impossible.

For treatment of acute symptomatology or in patients unable or unwilling to take oral medication, the usual dose is 4 mg of Navane (thiothixene hydrochloride) Intramuscular administered 2 to 4 times daily. Dosage may be increased or decreased depending on response. Most patients are controlled on a total daily dosage of 16 to 20 mg. The maximum recommended dosage is 30 mg/day. An oral form should supplant the injectable form as soon as possible. It may be necessary to adjust the dosage when changing from the intramuscular to oral dosage forms. Dosage recommendations for Navane Capsules and Concentrate can be found in the Navane oral package insert.

OVERDOSAGE. Manifestations include muscular twitching, drowsiness, and dizziness. Symptoms of gross overdosage may include CNS depression, rigidity, weakness, torticollis, tremor, salivation, dysphagia, hypotension, disturbances of gait, or coma.

Treatment: Essentially symptomatic and supportive. Keep patient under careful observation and maintain an open airway, since involvement of the extrapyramidal system may produce dysphagia and respiratory difficulty in severe overdosage. If hypotension occurs, the standard measures for managing circulatory shock should be used (I.V. fluids and/or vasoconstrictors).

If a vasoconstrictor is needed, levarterenol and phenylephrine are the most suitable drugs. Other pressor agents, including epinephrine, are not recommended, since phenothiazine derivatives may reverse the usual pressor elevating action of these agents and cause further lowering of blood pressure.

If CNS depression is present, recommended stimulants include amphetamine, dextroamphetamine, or caffeine and sodium benzoate. Picrotoxin or pentylenetetrazol should be avoided. Extrapyramidal symptoms may be treated with antiparkinson drugs.

There are no data on the use of peritoneal or hemodialysis, but they are known to be of little value in phenothiazine intoxication.

HOW SUPPLIED. Navane (thiothixene hydrochloride) Intramuscular Solution is available in a 2 ml amber glass vial in packages of 10 vials. Each ml contains thiothixene hydrochloride equivalent to 2 mg of thiothixene, dextrose 5% w/v, benzyl alcohol 0.9% w/v, and propyl gallate 0.02% w/v.

Navane Intramuscular For Injection is available in amber glass vials in packages of 10 vials. When reconstituted with 2.2 ml of Sterile Water for Injection, each ml contains thiothixene hydrochloride equivalent to 5 mg of thiothixene, and 59.6 mg of mannitol. The reconstituted solution of Navane Intramuscular For Injection may be stored for 48 hours at room temperature before discarding.

Emergency Psychiatry for the House Officer

Emergency Psychiatry for the House Officer

William R. Dubin, M.D.
Department of Psychiatry
Jefferson Crisis Service
Thomas Jefferson Medical University
Philadelphia, Pennsylvania

and

Robert Stolberg, M.D.
Department of Psychiatry
University of Puerto Rico School of Medicine
San Juan, Puerto Rico

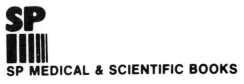

SP MEDICAL & SCIENTIFIC BOOKS

New York

SPECTRUM PUBLICATIONS, INC.
175-20 Wexford Terrace, Jamaica, N.Y.11432

Library of Congress Cataloging in Publication Data

Dubin, William R.
  Emergency psychiatry for the House Officer

  Includes index
  1. Psychiatric emergencies. I. Stolberg, Robert.
II. Title [DNLM: 1. Crisis intervention.
2. Emergency services, Hospital. 3. Mental disorders—
Therapy. 4. Mental health services. WM 401 D814c]
RC480.6.D8   616.89'025   81-40519
ISBN 0-89335-149-0   AACR2

second printing

This book is dedicated with love to our wives
Alicia and Glorisa
and our sons,
Brian David and Juan Carlos

Acknowledgments

We wish to express our gratitude to Dr. Roy Clouse for his help and encouragement in the preparation of this manuscript; to Drs. Neil Dubin, Joseph Zeccardi, Marc Rothman, Thomas Benfield and Greg Hyle for their helpful suggestions in preparing the manuscript, and to Dr. Alan Frazer for his encouragement in publishing the book.

We are especially indebted to Drs. Eli Marcovitz, the late Albert Biele, Paul Fink, Howard Field and the late Keith F. Sanders for the influence that they have had academically and professionally in shaping our careers.

We would like to express our appreciation to our parents, Sylvia and Sidney Dubin and Harry and Josefina Stolberg, for their love and guidance.

Finally we would like to thank Ailsa Kercadó, Vivian L. Nieves, Emelis D. Pérez, Syndi Cave, Pat Klevens, Michelle Johnson and Connie Baylor for their tireless efforts in typing the manuscript.

Preface

In the course of our work in emergency psychiatry at Thomas Jefferson University Hospital we found that there were no books that provided the houseofficer with a concise, practical guide to the management of psychiatric emergencies. Based on our own experiences we wrote *Emergency Psychiatry for the Houseofficer* with the idea of providing treatment principles that would allow non-psychiatric physicians and psychiatric residents to evaluate and provide interim treatment for a period of about 6 hours. We do not claim that this book is a comprehensive guide to psychiatry; instead our approach is problem oriented and the book is designed for easy, rapid reference in emergency situations.

William R. Dubin, M.D.
Robert Stolberg, M.D.

Contents

Chapter 1
Introduction

Introduction

Psychiatric patients can be among the most disconcerting patients to treat in an emergency department setting. Because these patients often present with violence, confusion, suicidal attempts and bizarre behavior and thoughts, non-psychiatric physicians often react with various degrees of discomfort and avoidance. However, it is often important to make a decision whether the presenting symptoms are due to functional or organic illness since serious morbidity and mortality can occur in patients with acute organic brain disease. The differential diagnosis would include:

Functional (Psychiatric) Disease

    Affective Disorders
    Schizophrenic Disorders
    Personality Disorders
    Anxiety Disorders
    Adjustment Disorders

Organic Disease

    Delirium
    Dementia

Findings which are helpful in raising the index of suspicion for organic disease are:

a)   Disorientation to time and place
b)   Fluctuating levels of consciousness

c) Age over 45 with no previous psychiatric history
d) Abnormal autonomic signs (vital signs, pupillary responses, sweating)
e) Acute onset of psychotic illness (hours to days)
f) Ongoing medical disease and its treatment
g) Recognition that hallucinations and delusions are frequently observed in organic as well as functional disease.

A thorough physical and psychiatric examination along with appropriate laboratory tests will usually provide the examiner with enough information to determine whether the patient is suffering from functional or organic disease. An understanding of the following basic terminology is necessary for consistency in the assessment of psychiatric patients:

A. Delirium—Sometimes delirium and acute organic brain syndrome (OBS) are used synonymously to define conditions of impaired brain function characterized by reversibility. Generally the patient presents with some or all of the following findings:

1. fluctuating levels of consciousness
2. disorientation
3. apprehension and fear
4. autonomic dysfunctions
5. agitation—may or may not be present
6. incoherence   In the presence of these symptoms
7. hallucinations   acute OBS can be mistaken for
8. illusions   functional psychiatric illness by the
9. delusions   unwary.

In general, delirium results from toxic, metabolic or systemic illnesses. It is usually present for several days at most and clears with resolution of the primary disorder. Examples of delirious behavior can be found in patients with sepsis, hypoxia, uremia, electrolyte imbalance, alcohol withdrawal, and various drug intoxications.

B. Dementia is a clinical syndrome marked most characteristically by chronicity and by impairment of all cognitive functions (perceiving, thinking, remembering). It differs from delirium in that patients with dementia do not have fluctuating levels of consciousness, are generally not agitated, and may have had intellectual impairment for a considerable period of time. Early symptoms are likely to be vague or to suggest a more functional psychiatric disease.

Early symptoms include:

1. somatic complaints
2. depression and anxiety
3. irritability
4. mild memory loss
5. diminished drive and creativity
6. declining interest in former activities and hobbies
7. increased difficulty in adapting to new circumstances
8. lack of perseverance in tasks

These symptoms are usually insidious and recognized only in retrospect.

Middle phase: The symptoms that occur in this phase are generally the symptoms that result in the patient being brought to the physician for an evaluation and include:

1. impairment of memory
2. impairment of orientation
3. impairment of judgment
4. impairment of all intellectual functions
5. lability and shallowness of mood

Late phase:

1. apathy
2. neurologic impairment predominates

Old age itself does not cause dementia. "Senility" is not an acceptable neurological term. Senility would imply that old age is a disease and also that old age is the cause of disease, especially intellectual impairment. At no age is dementia a normal state of affairs and despite the chronic aspect of dementia, *in many cases it is reversible.* Dementia has multiple etiologies and senile dementia is diagnosed only after all other causes are ruled out.

C. Psychosis is characterized by a severe degree of personality disorganization. This disorganization affects the patient so that he is generally unable to deal realistically with everyday living, i.e., work, school, marriage, interpersonal relationships. Psychosis can result from disordered thought and perceptions (schizophrenia), alteration in mood (affective disorders), or impairment of sensorium and cognition (delirium). Psychotic patients may also manifest poor impulse control, childlike behavior, hallucinations, delusions, and illusions. Psychosis, like anemia, implies a general nonspecific medical condition which requires a thorough medical and psychiatric evaluation for diagnosis before definitive treatment can begin.

D. Personality disorders refer to a group of disorders which result from an individual's maladaptive pattern of behavior. Personality generally describes a person's characteristic patterns of behavior and responses to the environment and other people. A personality disorder reflects a developmental problem which has resulted in a flaw in the patient's personality so that his mode of relating to other people and the environment is maladaptive. A personality disorder is generally of long standing duration and may be recognized by an individual's chronic difficulty with personal relationships, difficulties with jobs, repeated legal difficulties, or recognizable eccentricities. Types of personality disorders include: explosive, histrionic, borderline, antisocial, paranoid. Patients with personality disorders are difficult to treat because they view their behavior and attitudes as an acceptable part of their total personality.

E. Situational disturbances occur generally in patients secondary to an overwhelming, definable environmental stress. The disturbance may range from mild symptoms such as insomnia and anxiousness to overt psychosis. The disturbance is time-limited and remission will occur with removal of the stress.

F. Anxiety disorders are a group of disorders in which the chief manifestations are physical symptoms and a sense of impending doom. These disorders may reflect an underlying medical illness or the disorders may be purely functional and represent the patient's unconscious fears of losing control of his impulses, fears of separation, or fears of punishment. Generally, the patient is not aware of the psychological dynamics which form the basis for the anxiety.

References

1. Anderson, William. Emergency Department, in *Handbook of General Hospital Psychiatry*, edited by Hackett and Cassem, C.V. Mosby Co., St. Louis, Missouri, 1978, pp. 392–404.
2. *Diagnostic and Statistical Manual of Mental Disorders*, Third Edition, American Psychiatric Association, Washington, D.C., 1980.
3. Kolb, Lawrence C. Senile and Presenile Psychoses in *Modern Clinical Psychiatry*. W.B. Saunders Co., Philadelphia, Pa., 1977, pp. 183–195.
4. Lipowski, Z.J. Delirium, Clouding of Consciousness, and Confusion. *Journal of Nervous and Mental Disease*, 145:227–255, 1967.
5. Wells, Charles E. Chronic Brain Disease: An Overview. *American Journal of Psychiatry*, 135:1–12, 1978.
6. Wells, Charles E. and Duncan, Gary W. *Neurology for Psychiatrists*. F.A. Davis Co., Philadelphia, 1980.
7. *A Psychiatric Glossary*, American Psychiatric Association (Publications Office, 1700 18th Street, N.W.), Washington, D.C.

Chapter 2
The Psychiatric Examination

Introduction

The psychiatric examination involves the systematic collection of data about the patient in order to make an appropriate diagnosis. A complete psychiatric evaluation includes the following: present illness, past psychiatric and medical treatment, marital history, education, occupational history, social history (e.g., use of drugs, alcohol, relationships with other people) and a mental status examination. Especially with men, it is also helpful to ask about their service record, e.g., type of discharge, demotions, etc. A complete examination always includes a physical and neurological evaluation since patients with organic disease frequently present with predominantly behavioral abnormalities in the emergency department. When psychiatric patients are unable to give an adequate history, the interviewer should attempt to contact family or friends for a more complete history.

The assessment of the current mental functioning of the patient is of special importance and is referred to as the mental status examination. In the emergency department, the mental status evaluation is an indispensable guide to separating delirium and dementia from the functional psychoses. The mental status is used to evaluate orientation, memory, fund of knowledge, and to determine the presence of a thinking or affective disorder. In most cases, the mental status of the patient can be assessed from the clinical interview. In the uncooperative, acutely

7

disturbed patient, observable mental-status findings such as appearance, behavior, speech, and emotional expression can often provide enough information to establish a working diagnosis.

The mental status can be divided into ten broad areas: appearance, behavior, speech, thought process and content, perception, affect, sensorium, cognitive functioning, insight and judgment. In evaluating the mental status of a patient, it is helpful to remember that psychiatric diagnosis is not based on pathognomonic symptoms but is based on a cluster of symptoms and a longitudinal history which characterizes specific syndromes.

Mental Status Evaluation

The mental status is the assessment of how a person is functioning at a given point in time. The clinician collects clinical and/or observable data as follows (see Table I):

A. Appearance: Within the first few minutes of contact with the patient, the physician can start to collect considerable clinical data, a great deal of which initially pertains to appearance.

1. Attire and bodily care may give a clue to a patient's ability to care for his well-being or the appropriateness of his judgment.
   a) neat and well-groomed: suggestive of a non-psychotic illness.
   b) disheveled and unkempt: suggestive of schizophrenia, depression, alcohol or drug abuse.
   c) bizarre and eccentric: suggestive of schizophrenia or at times mania.
   d) careless, indifferent: suggestive of depression, drug or alcohol abuse.

B. Behavior: The behavior of a patient includes observable body movements and posture. Examples of disordered behavior include:

1. Tremors (fine and coarse), pill rolling: suggestive of anxiety, medication side effects, alcohol withdrawal.

2. Agitation (pacing, restlessness, generalized motor excitement):

suggestive of mania, schizophrenia, drug intoxication (amphetamine), alcohol withdrawal, anxiety.

3. Motor retardation (slow initiation of movement):
   a) catatonic—extreme motor retardation with immobility. At times catatonia may present as extreme motor excitement: suggestive of schizophrenia, depression, mania.
   b) waxy flexibility—maintaining body position in which it is placed: suggestive of schizophrenia.

4. Carpologia—aimless picking, plucking of clothes or bed covering: suggestive of delirium, dementia.

5. Echopraxia—imitation of movement and gestures of interviewer: suggestive of chronic schizophrenia, dementia, or delirium.

6. Apraxia—loss of ability to complete voluntary goal—directed movements: suggestive of neurologic disease.

7. Extrapyramidal symptoms: suggestive of neuroleptic side effects.
   a) akathisia—feeling of restlessness or compelling need for movement.
   b) akinesia—absence or loss of the power of voluntary action.
   c) dyskinesia—facial grimacing, perioral movements or tongue protrusion. Involuntary choreiform movements of limbs may occur.
   d) Parkinsonian effects—muscular rigidity, fine, resting tremor.

C. Speech

1. Rate of speech
   a) mutism—refusal to speak: suggestive of schizophrenia, depression.
   b) retardation—a marked slowness of initiation and rate of speech—suggestive of depression.
   c) pressure of speech—rapid, uninterruptible speech: suggestive of mania or extreme anxiety.
   d) slurred speech: suggestive of drug or alcohol intoxication.
   e) aphasia—a disorder of speech which results in difficulties in the comprehension and expression of words: suggestive of dementia.

TABLE I Suggestive Indicators of Common Psychiatric Syndromes

Mental Status	Schizophrenia	Mania	Depression	Delirium	Dementia
Appearance	Bizarre, eccentric, disheveled	Varies from well dressed to disheveled, eccentric	Careless, indifferent, stooped posture, depressed facies	Non-specific	Non-specific
Behavior	Bizarre, withdrawn, occasionally agitated	Hyperactive, restless, gregarious, amusing	Motor retardation, tearful, may present agitated	Agitated, restless. At times, agitation absent, and patient is "quietly delirious," carpologia	Lethargic, apathetic, apraxia, echopraxia
Speech	Mute, bizarre, rambling, incoherent	Rapid, pressured	Speech retarded, in monotone	Non-specific	Echolalia, aphasia
Thought	Loose associations, thought blocking, persecutory, bizarre, grandiose delusions, ideas of reference	Flight of ideas, may have grandiose or paranoid delusions	Ideas of helplessness and hopelessness, suicidal ideation, possible delusions of poverty, guilt, sin	Circumstantial, delusions, ability to reason is impaired, ideas of reference	Perseveration, inability to abstract, occasionally disorganized delusions

Perception	Hallucinations	Hallucinations may occur	Hallucinations uncommon	Illusions, hallucinations	—
Affect	Flat, inappropriate	Elation, frequently irritable	Sad, downcast, despondent	Labile	Labile
Cognition	Orientation* memory intact*	Orientation* memory intact*	Orientation* memory intact*	Disoriented, impaired memory	Disoriented, impaired memory
Physical findings	—	—	—	Abnormal autonomic signs, fluctuating consciousness, tremors, pupillary changes	Frontal lobe release signs, corticospinal tract abnormalities

*May appear to be impaired by patient's inability to attend and by patient's distractibility.

2. Unusual disordered speech: suggestive of chronic schizophrenia or organic brain disease.
    a) neologism—new term created by condensation of unrelated words which has special meaning to the patient.
    b) word salad—incoherent mixture of words and phrases.
    c) echolalia—repetition of another person's words or phrases.
    d) perseveration—repetition of a word, phrase or idea to varied stimuli.

D. Thought Process

1. Thought processes reflect the coherence of the flow of ideas.
    a) circumstantiality—patient reaches a goal after numerous unnecessary digressions: suggestive of chronic schizophrenia, organic brain disease, or obsessive personality.
    b) flight of ideas—rapid succession of thoughts that are context-bound, i.e., connected with each other or with the environment in a way that can usually be understood: suggestive of mania.
    c) looseness of association—succession of thoughts that are not context-bound, i.e., the examiner can not detect any connection between them or with the environment: suggestive of schizophrenia.
    d) clang associations—thoughts merely associated by words similar in sound but not significance (lawyer-liar): suggestive of mania, schizophrenia.
    e) obsessive thinking—insistent thoughts which repetitively recur and which the patient cannot keep out of his mind: suggestive of obsessive–compulsive disorder.
    f) thought blocking—sudden cessation of thought: suggestive of schizophrenia.

E. Thought Content is concerned with the ideas that make up the patient's thoughts.

1. Delusion—a fixed, false belief which is not consistent with logic but is maintained despite all rational evidence against the belief. Delusions may consist of several types, including:

a) delusion of persecution, or grandeur: suggestive of schizophrenia or mania.
b) delusion of religiosity: suggestive of schizophrenia.
c) delusion of guilt, poverty, nihilism: suggestive of depression.
d) somatic delusion: suggestive of depression, schizophrenia.

2. Ideas of reference—the belief that other people are talking about or referring to the patient by means of gestures or smiles: suggestive of schizophrenia, psychotic depression, alcohol withdrawal.

3. Suicidal thoughts—preoccupation with killing oneself: suggestive of depression, personality disorder.

4. Homicidal thoughts—preoccupation with killing someone: suggestive of psychosis, personality disorder.

F. Perception

1. Misperceptions may consist of:
   a) illusions— a false interpretation of a real sensory stimulus: suggestive of delirium.
   b) hallucinations — a false perception without any sensory stimulus. Hallucinations include several types:
      (1) Auditory hallucinations: suggestive of schizophrenia or alcoholic hallucinosis.
      (2) Visual hallucinations: suggestive of delirium, alcohol withdrawal, drug intoxication. (To differentiate organic from psychogenic hallucinations, see Table II.)
      (3) Olfactory hallucinations: suggestive of a frontal or temporal lobe lesion, epilepsy.
      (4) Tactile hallucinations: suggestive of delirium, schizophrenia.
      (5) Gustatory hallucinations: suggestive of a frontal or temporal lobe lesion, epilepsy.

G. Emotional Expression: This is the most difficult facet of the mental status to assess with clinical objectivity. It includes:

1. Mood—feeling, tone experienced internally by the patient.

TABLE II A Comparison of Organic and Psychogenic Visual Hallucinations (Biele, 1974)

Organic	Psychogenic
a. Sharply demarcated	a. Vague, shadowy, misty
b. Vivid and well-formed	b. Usually in shades of gray
c. Polychromic and/or poly-sonic	c. Fleeting, transient
d. Hypermobility, i.e., bugs creeping, elephants stampeding	d. May be associated with patient's psychodynamics
e. Accompanied by terror, apprehension	e. Patient has an *idea* that he sees, feels, but does not really see, feel the hallucinated subject.
f. Perseverative quality	
g. Patient *acts* as though he really sees, hears, feels, etc.	

2. Affect—the outward manifestation of a feeling that is attached to an object, idea or thought. Examples of affect include:
   a) Fear
   b) Rage
   c) Pleasure
   d) Depression
   e) Elation
   f) Anxiety

3. Unusual emotional tones
   a) Inappropriate affect—lack of harmony between expression of feeling tone and thoughts (for example, a patient laughs over sad event): suggestive of schizophrenia.
   b) Flat affect—expressionless speech and facies regardless of idea, subject, or thought: suggestive of schizophrenia.
   c) La belle indifference—lack of concern about a disability: suggestive of conversion disorder.
   d) Lability of affect—unstable, rapidly changing emotions within seconds: suggestive of delirium, dementia.
   e) Euphoria—a sense of emotional and physical well-being not

justified by circumstances: suggestive of mania, drug or alcohol intoxication.

H. Sensorium and Cognitive Functioning: These tests are useful in differentiating functional from organic illness. Defects in the various spheres of orientation, memory and general information are suggestive of delirium, dementia, or drug and alcohol intoxication or withdrawal.

1. Orientation—patient's orientation is usually lost sequentially for *time* (date, month, year) and then *place* (where he is), and very rarely for *person.*

2. Memory—performance is influenced by intelligence, age, depression, or anxiety. Tests helpful in assessing memory include:
   a) Recall of recent and remote events
   b) Repetition of three objects in five minutes
   c) General information such as patient's home address, names of children and their ages, mayor of city, president of United States, etc.

3. Attention and concentration—is measured by subtraction of serial numbers starting from 100. This primarily measures capacity to sustain effort on a given task.

4. Calculation—is performed by simple addition, subtraction, multiplication, and division. Errors are usually secondary to disorders of attention, concentration or intelligence, except for the very rare syndrome of dyscalculia seen in Gerstmann's Syndrome, a disorder of small dominant parietal lobe lesion.

5. Abstraction tests—similarities between two items; meaning of proverbs. Influenced by intelligence, anxiety, socioeconomic background. It is useful for general exploration of the thought processes. It helps at times to detect looseness of association or unusual preoccupations.

6. Judgment—is the awareness of the consequences of intended behavior. Ability to maintain good judgment is dependent on intact consciousness, orientation, memory, attention and concentration.

7. Insight—reflects the extent to which the patient is aware that he is ill and has symptoms that impair his usual state of effective functioning.

Medical Evaluation

In addition to the history and mental status exam, physical and neurological examinations are also necessary in acutely psychotic patients in order to rule out delirium, drug or alcohol intoxication and withdrawal.

A. Physical Examination: There are certain parts of the physical examination which can be helpful in determining the presence of organic disease. These include:

1. Levels of consciousness—altered levels of consciousness suggest organic disease, drug or alcohol abuse.
    a) Awake and clear: fully aware of surroundings
    b) Awake but confused as to where he is
    c) Stuporous: can be aroused by vigorous shaking or calling of name, but relapses back into unconsciousness
    d) Coma
       (1) Grade I—Responds to painful stimuli.
                    Deep tendon reflexes are present.
                    Vital signs are stable.
       (2) Grade II—Does not respond to painful stimuli.
                    Deep tendon reflexes are present.
                    Vital signs are stable.
       (3) Grade III—Does not respond to painful stimuli.
                    Deep tendon reflexes are not present.
                    Vital signs are stable.
       (4) Grade IV—Does not respond to painful stimuli.
                    Deep tendon reflexes are not present.
                    Vital signs are not stable and support of blood pressure and respiration is required.

2. Vital signs and autonomic signs: when abnormal, suggests toxic/

metabolic encephalopathy.
a) Temperature
b) Pulse
c) Blood pressure
d) Respirations
e) Sweating
f) Dryness of mouth
g) Absence of bowel sounds
h) Pupillary responses
 (1) Dilated, Reactive—amphetamine intoxication
 (2) Dilated, Non-reactive—atropine intoxication
 (3) Constricted—suggests narcotic intoxication, pontine lesion
 (4) Nystagmus, somnolence and ataxia—suggests barbiturate intoxication

3. Fundi—papilledema is evidence of increased intercranial pressure.

4. Skull—laceration or a depression of the skull suggests head trauma.

5. Ears—blood or cerebral spinal fluid around the tympanic membranes can provide evidence of a basilar skull fracture.

6. Tremor, Asterixis—suggests hepatic failure, renal failure, thyrotoxicosis, impending D.T.'s.

B. Neurological Examination

1. Salient features of the neurological examination of patients with altered mental status.
 a) Signs of structural neurological disease
  (1) Focal or lateralizing findings
  (2) Papilledema
 b) Neurological findings associated with dementia
  (1) Frontal lobe release signs, snout, suck and rooting reflexes, grasp, and palmarmental reflexes
  (2) Apraxis, aphasia
  (3) Corticospinal tract abnormalities such as spastic paresis, hyperactive tendon reflexes, a positive Babinski response.

References

1. Anderson, W.H. The Physical Examination in Office Practice. *American Journal of Psychiatry,* 137:1188–1192, 1980.
2. Bannister, Roger. *Brain's Clinical Neurology,* 4th Edition. Oxford University Press, London, 1973.
3. Biele, A.M. *The Mental Status Examination* (unpublished manuscript), 1974.
4. Bensen, F.D., and Blumer, D., editors. *Psychiatric Aspects of Neurologic Disease,* Grune and Stratton, New York, 1975.
5. Eysenck, J.J. and Halstead, H. The Memory Function, A functional study of fifteen clinical tests. *American Journal of Psychiatry,* 102: 174–180, 1945.
6. Freeman, Thomas. *Psychopathology of the Psychoses,* International Universities Press, New York, 1969.
7. Hamilton, Max. *Fish's Clinical Psychopathology,* John Wright and Sons, Bristol, England, 1974.
8. Hinton, J. and Withers, E. The Usefulness of the Clinical Tests of the Sensorium. *British Journal of Psychiatry,* 119:9–18, 1971.
9. Lishman, William Alwyn. *Organic Psychiatry,* Blackwell Scientific Publications, London, 1978.
10. Milstein, V., Small, J. and Small, I. The Substraction of Serial Seven Test in Psychiatric Patients. *Archives of General Psychiatry,* 26:439–441, 1972.
11. Nathan, P.E. Differential Diagnostic Symptoms and Signs Chapter 6, in *Handbook of Psychiatry,* edited by Philip Solomon and Vernon D. Patch, Lange Medical Publication, Los Altos, California, 1974, pp. 86–100.
12. Setter, J.G. Treatment of Acute CNS Depressant Emergencies in *A Treatment Manual for Acute Drug Abuse Emergencies,* edited by Peter G. Bourne, U.S. Department of Health, Education, and Welfare, Rockville, Maryland, 1976.
13. Smith, A. The Serial Sevens Subtraction Test. *Archives of Neurology,* 17:78–80, 1967.
14. Weiner, H.L., and Levitt, L.P. *Neurology for the House Officer,* 2nd edition, Williams and Wilkins Co., Baltimore, 1978.
15. Wells, Charles E. and Duncan, Gary W. *Neurology for Psychiatrists,* F.A. Davis Co., Philadelphia, 1980.
16. Withers, E. and Hinton, I. Three forms of the clinical test of the sensorium and their reliability. *British Journal of Psychiatry,* 119: 18, 1971.
17. *A Psychiatric Glossary,* 4th edition, American Psychiatric Association (Publication Office, 1700 Eighteenth Street, N.W.), Washington, D.C.

Chapter 3

Organic Brain Syndromes –
Delirium and Dementia

Delirium

The ability of the physician to recognize delirium in the emergency department is critical, since irreversible brain damage or death can occur in unrecognized cases. Because patients with delirium frequently exhibit predominantly confused, bizarre activity or act in a belligerent, agitated manner, they are often misdiagnosed as having a functional illness and are referred to a psychiatrist after a cursory physical examination. Four factors which suggest delirium include:

A. Disorientation
B. Fluctuating consciousness
C. A patient over age 45 with no previous psychiatric history
D. Abnormal autonomic signs

In the presence of any one of these four findings, the examining physician must consider delirium, dementia, alcohol or drug intoxication or withdrawal, and begin a physical and laboratory diagnostic evaluation. Although alcohol intoxications and withdrawals are considered organic brain syndromes, we will deal with these in separate chapters.

I. EVALUATION

Delirium is a result of transient brain dysfunction and generally manifests behavioral abnormalities as part of the symptom complex. The diagnosis is based on clinical features, history, physical and laboratory findings.

A. The clinical presentation can include:

1. Disorientation to time, place and person.

2. Memory impairment—occurs in variable degrees in both recent and/or remote spheres.

3. Fluctuating consciousness—e.g., the patient's state of consciousness fluctuates between alertness, confusion, stupor and, sometimes, coma.

4. Labile affect—e.g., the patient can quickly change from being pleasant to being angry, from belligerence to friendliness.

5. Impaired judgment and insight.

6. Hallucinations—are generally visual, vivid, and usually in color. The hallucinations change rapidly and are not consistent throughout the course of the examination, e.g., the patient might initially hallucinate that a truck is driving through his examining room, and a few minutes later the patient might hallucinate that a foreign army is invading. Auditory hallucinations generally occur in schizophrenia, while visual hallucinations generally occur in delirium.

7. Delusions—like hallucinations, delusions may also change rapidly.

8. Illusions—delirious patients frequently will misinterpret sensory stimuli, e.g., the crack in the wall is perceived as a snake.

9. Agitation—the patient may be restless, hyperactive, tremulous. In contrast, a patient may also experience a "quiet delirium" in which he appears to be resting comfortably and only on close examination will the physician find that the patient is disoriented and hallucinating with marked memory impairment.

10. Frequently the symptoms of delirium worsen at night. This phenomenon is referred to as the "sundowners' syndrome."

11. Disturbance of the sleep/wakefulness cycle with insomnia or daytime drowsiness.

12. Difficulty sustaining attention and easily distracted by irrelevant stimuli.

In the presence of the above symptoms delirium must be suspected. Remember, *most* patients who have schizophrenic or affective disorders do not show memory impairment, disorientation, or fluctuating levels of consciousness.

B. History and physical evaluation: Evaluation includes complete medical history and physical examination (see Chapter 2). Delirium can occur at any age. The onset is usually abrupt (hours to days) and the course fluctuates with periods of lucidity and confusion.

C. Laboratory evaluation: The laboratory evaluation is an integral part of the workup for delirium and dementia and should include:

1. Complete Blood Count (CBC) and differential*

2. Urinalysis*

3. Glucose, BUN, Electrolytes*

4. EKG*

5. Chest X-ray*

6. SMA 12-chemistry profile of renal and hepatic status (LDH, SGOT, total Bilirubin, Creatinine, Uric acid, total protein, Albumin)

7. VDRL

8. Thyroid function tests

9. Sedimentation rate

10. Fluorescent antinuclear antibody

*May be done in the emergency department

11. B12 level

12. Folic acid level

13. EEG

D. Additional neurological diagnostic procedures include:

1. The Skull x-ray will usually demonstrate only calcified tumors, shifts of a calcified pineal gland and signs of increased intracranial pressure. The x-ray will be normal in most cases of cerebral mass lesions as well as toxic metabolic and degenerative disease. Patients with abnormal findings on skull x-rays will usually have florid clinical abnormalities. Therefore, a skull x-ray is an inappropriate screening device because it is normal in almost all cases of OBS and abnormal only when advanced neurological disease is present. Generally used when history or evidence of head trauma is present.

2. The EEG is useful in detecting alterations in neurological function. It will be abnormal with diseases such as neoplastic, vascular, degenerative and toxic-metabolic and seizure disorders. Certain diseases besides epilepsy have characteristic electroencephalographic patterns, e.g., Jacob Creutzfeldt and subacute sclerosing panencephalitis (SSPE). Unfortunately, the EEG may be abnormal with trivial conditions such as lethargy, older age and use of many medications. As a screening device the EEG is excellent. An EEG is required as part of a thorough evaluation.

3. The Isotopic Brain Scan's sole use is in detection of cerebral mass lesions, i.e., neoplasms, abscess, hematoma, contusion, infarction and vascular malformations, which it is able to do with greater reliability than either the EEG or skull x-rays. Of course, it will not detect metabolic or physiological disturbances. If lateralizing signs are present or if there is a focal EEG abnormality, the brain scan is indicated. In the near future it will be replaced by computerized tomography as a screening device for cerebral mass lesions.

4. Computed tomography (CT). The CT scan permits detection of cerebral lesions such as tumors, infarctions and congenital

abnormalities. It will also detect cerebral atrophy, brain edema, and hydrocephalus. Metabolic physiological disturbances will re-remain undetected. The CT is an excellent diagnostic procedure for patients with dementia or signs of focal CNS disease and is preferred to the brain scan.

5. Cerebral angiography is useful in diagnosis of intracranial vascular thrombosis, hemorrhage, brain abscess, neoplasm, atherosclerotic plaques, and occlusions which may be causing a progressive OBS.

6. The examination of cerebrospinal fluid (CSF) by lumbar puncture might reveal evidence of nervous system infections which cause dementia, such as fungal meningitis, syphilis and encephalitis. It might also provide evidence of neoplastic disease and subarachnoid hemorrhage. The LP is necessary in the complete evaluation of cases of delirium and dementia since it is the only test which might detect evidence of CNS infection. It is frequently not performed unless there is an abnormal EEG or evidence of systemic infection or cerebral vascular accident. Prior to doing a lumbar puncture, the examiner should check the fundi, for evidence of increased intracranial pressure.

E. Further special tests
   Heavy metal screening (lead and mercury)
   Bromide screening (if serum chloride evaluated)
   Urine for porphyrins (Porphyria)
   Serum ceruploplasm (Wilson's Disease)
   CSF measles antibodies (if subacute sclerosing encephalitis is suspected)

With judicious use, these tests should serve as an adequate screen for structural lesions, toxic and metabolic disorders and infectious processes. The combination of a thorough examination, general laboratory tests and neurological laboratory tests will usually indicate the general cause of the delirium or dementia and, more importantly, screen for all correctable causes of delirium and dementia.

II. There are several medical illnesses which commonly present as acute organic brain syndrome in the emergency department and should be recognized immediately in order to avoid irreversible brain damage and, in some instances, death. These include:

A. Hypoglycemia—Any patient who comes in with stupor or coma should immediately have a serum glucose determination and be given a bolus of 50 cc of 50% dextrose and water.

B. Diabetic ketosis and non-ketotic hyperosmolarity—In a known diabetic, the presence of delirium accompanied by hyperpnea, odor of acetone on the breath, dehydration, and hypotension, point to a diagnosis of diabetic ketosis. If hyperglycemia, glucosuria, and ketosuria are present, this establishes the diagnosis. Marked hyperglycemia and glucosuria in the absence of ketosuria make the diagnosis of nonketotic hyperosmolarity likely. Insulin plus intravenous saline is the emergency treatment of choice for both conditions, with further fluid replacement being determined by the monitoring of blood electrolytes and acid-base balance.

C. Wernicke-Korsakoff's Syndrome—should be suspected in any patient with a history of alcohol use who has nystagmus, cerebellar ataxia and evidence of peripheral neuropathy. Thiamine 100 mg intramuscularly should be given immediately.

D. Delirium tremens—is a diagnosis that is frequently missed and should be suspected in any patient with elevated autonomic signs, agitation, visual hallucinations, hyperreflexia and a history of alcohol abuse. The onset of delirium tremens is usually 3 to 4 days after the reduction of alcohol intake or after total abstinence.

E. Cerebral hypoxia—which can result from myocardial infarctions, pneumonia, chronic obstructive lung disease, and arrhythmias. It is a frequent cause of delirium seen in the emergency room.

F. Meningitis—should be suspected in the presence of a stiff neck and a fever.

G. Anticholinergic Intoxication—secondary to abuse of tricyclic antidepressants or large overdoses of over-the-counter drugs that contain atropine. The patients will frequently present with flushing, tachycardia, rapid pulse, hypertension and dilated pupils which are nonreactive or only sluggishly reactive to light. Most fatalities are caused by cardiac arrhythmias and the treatment of choice for atropine poisoning is physostigmine, 1 to 2 mgs. I.V. This may be repeated every 15 minutes as necessary to treat seizures, arrhythmias and coma. (With tricyclic antidepressants, a QRS duration of 100 milliseconds or greater can be used to define a major overdose.)

H. Subarachnoid hemorrhage—should be suspected in the presence of a stiff neck, fluctuating consciousness, complaint of headaches. A spinal tap should be done immediately.

I. Subdural hematoma—should be suspected in patients presenting with fluctuating consciousness and a history of head trauma. Subdural hematomas are common in alcoholics and the elderly.

J. Myocardial infarction—may cause cerebral hypoxia which will frequently result in behavioral abnormalities. Should be considered in all patients over 40 with no previous psychiatric history.

III. The most important aspect in diagnosing organic brain syndrome is to *think* organic brain syndrome and not make the assumption that every patient with bizarre behavior or every patient who is belligerent and agitated is a "psych" patient. Other common causes of acute organic brain syndrome which are commonly referred to the psychiatrist in an emergency room setting after being "medically cleared" include:

1. Pneumonia
2. Post-ictal states
3. Dilantin toxicity
4. Impending delirium tremens
5. Renal failure
6. Chronic obstructive lung disease

IV. One common cause of aberrant behavior is drug-induced delirium or psychosis in patients treated with medical drugs for systemic illness. Appendix I gives a detailed listing of the psychiatric side effects of medical drugs reproduced from the book *Psychiatric Presentation of Medical Illness* (Hall, 1980). In any patient being treated with drugs for medical illness, the drugs have to be considered as an etiology for the behavioral/psychological aberrations.

V. Treatment—The definitive treatment of delirium is to treat the underlying medical etiology. However, the psychological care of the delirious patient is important since it is frequently necessary to keep the patient from harming himself or others.

The patient should be supervised closely by nurses and/or family members in order to protect the patient from harming himself. Because delirious patients are suggestible, a friendly, reassuring attitude will help to calm the patient. Patients should be placed in a moderately lighted room and the use of physical restraints should be minimal. Excessive and conflicting sensory stimuli should be eliminated. Medical personnel should be clearly identified and should always state why they are there and what they are doing. Because delirious patients are irritable, they should not be placed in a room with another agitated patient. Once the diagnosis of delirium is made, the patient should not be continuously questioned since this will only serve to further agitate him. All statements to the patient should be simple and concrete. Finally, because a delirious patient's judgment is impaired, the family should be involved in all important medical decisions. If the patient becomes a management problem (i.e., combative, belligerent, agitated) and should require medication, neuroleptic medication, except in cases of drug and alcohol withdrawal (see chapters VIII and IX), is the drug of choice. Treatment doses are determined empirically based on age, weight and degree of physical debilitation. Dose ranges include:

1. Navane (thiothixene) 2 to 10 mg, I.M. or concentrate, every 30 minutes.
2. Stelazine (trifluoperazine) 5 to 15 mg, I.M. or concentrate, every 30 minutes.
3. Haldol (haloperidol) 0.5 to 5 mg, I.M. or concentrate, every 30 minutes.

These drugs can be safely given every 30 minutes until the patient becomes tranquilized. The patient's blood pressure should be taken before each dose is given. An exception is atropine psychosis where physostigmine is the drug of choice.

VI. DISPOSITION

If a proper diagnosis is made, some patients with acute OBS can be observed and treated in the emergency department and sent home. These include patients that are post-ictal, Dilantin toxic, or patients that are intoxicated from alcohol and drugs. However, the bulk of delirious patients generally require further medical evaluation and treatment; therefore, admission to a medical unit is preferable. Patients with acute OBS should only be admitted to a psychiatric unit when they are too disruptive to be managed elsewhere. However, the decision to admit to a psychiatric unit should only be considered after the patient's response to neuroleptic medication has been determined in the emergency department.

VII. DEMENTIA

A. Diagnosis

A thorough diagnostic evaluation can identify treatable causes of dementia in 30-50% of the cases. Of these, approximately 15% are potentially reversible. It is a gross injustice to elderly patients to assume that they are suffering from "senile dementia" when their physical examination is normal. Senile dementia is a diagnosis of exclusion and only after all possible causes have been ruled out should the diagnosis be made. The diagnosis of dementia is based on a constellation of clinical signs, physical and laboratory evaluation and history. The signs and symptoms of dementia include:

1. A history of an *insidious, slowly progressive* disorder, e.g., chronicity

2. *Impairment of all cognitive* functions (perceiving, thinking, remembering)

3. Constriction of interests

4. Difficulty adapting to new circumstances

5.   Marked memory impairment

6.   Poor judgment and insight that may manifest as deterioration of social habits, intellect or changes in normal day-to-day activities

7.   Labile affect

8.   Impairment of orientation

9.   Symptoms frequently *worsen at night*

10. Loss of sphincter control

11. Apraxis aphasias, agnosias

12. There are usually no hallucinations, delusions, illusions, or fluctuations in consciousness.

B.   Laboratory Evaluation—The laboratory evaluation is the same as for delirium.

C.   The list of reversible and irreversible causes of dementia is quite extensive (Table I and II). There are certain reversible causes of dementia that the examining physician should remember (London, 1978). These include:

1.   Chronic subdural hematoma(s)

2.   Neurosyphilis

3.   Pernicious anemia (that is, combined systems disease)

4.   Vitamin deficiencies (Thiamine: Wernicke's encephalopathy and Korsakoff's psychosis; Niacin: pellagra, the 3 D's — dementia, diarrhea, dermatitis)

5.   Endocrine abnormality (of the thyroid, parathyroid or adrenal gland, and hypoglycemia)

6.   Depression (In the elderly, depression often presents as senility.)

7.   Drug-induced (alcohol, tranquilizers, over-the-counter preparations)

8.   Exogenous toxins (carbon monoxide, bromide, mercury, lead, etc.)

9. Metabolic abnormality (of cardiac, pulmonary, hepatic or renal origin, or of calcium or the electrolytes)

10. Excess copper (Wilson's disease)

11. Normal pressure hydrocephalus

12. Tumor (particularly a slow growing meningioma)

13. Infection (tuberculosis, herpes simplex encephalitis—now treatable with adenine arabinoside)

14. Hyponatremia (due to inappropriate ADH secretion)

A helpful mnemonic to remember reversible causes of dementia is "S_2AV_2E $D_2EMENTIA$"

TABLE I   Treatable Forms of Dementia (from Slaby, 1980)

1. Addison's Disease
2. Some angiomas of the cerebral vessels
3. Anoxia secondary to cardiac or respiratory disease
4. Cerebral abscess
5. Some cerebral neoplasias
6. Chronic subdural hematoma(s)
7. Electrolyte imbalance
8. Endogenous toxins (as with hepatic or renal failure)
9. Exogenous toxins such as carbon monoxide
10. Hypothyroidism
11. Hypoglycemia
12. Cerebral infections such as tuberculosis, syphilis, parasites or yeasts
13. Intracranial aneurysms
14. Normal-pressure hydrocephalus
15. Pseudodementia
16. Vitamin deficiencies
17. Wilson's disease

TABLE II Untreatable Forms of Dementia (from Slaby, 1980)

1. Alcoholic encephalopathy
2. Alzheimer's disease
3. Arteriosclerosis
4. Behcet's syndrome
5. Cerebral metastases
6. Some primary cerebral neoplasms
7. Creutzfeldt-Jakob's disease
8. Dementia pugilistica
9. Familiar myoclonus epilepsy
10. Friedreich's ataxia
11. Huntington's chorea
12. Kuf's disease
13. Marchiafava-Bignami disease
14. Down's syndrome
15. Multiple myeloma
16. Multiple sclerosis
17. Collagenous disease
18. Parkinsonism—dementia complex of Guam
19. Pick's disease
20. Post-concussion syndrome
21. Presenile dementia with motor neuron disease
22. Presenile glial dystrophy
23. Primary parenchymatous cerebellar atrophy with dementia
24. Primary subcortical gliosis
25. Progressive supranuclear palsy
26. Sarcoidiosis
27. Schilder's disease
28. Senile dementia
29. Trauma
30. Simple presenile dementia

TABLE III Clinical Features Differentiating Pseudodementia from Dementia (from Wells, 1978b)

Pseudodementia	Dementia
1. Symptoms usually of short duration	1. Symptoms usually of long duration
2. Patients usually complain much of cognitive loss	2. Patients often appear unaware of cognitive loss
3. Patients usually communicate strong feelings of distress	3. Patients often appear untroubled
4. Attention and concentration appear well-preserved	4. Attention and concentration usually defective
5. "Don't know" answers typical	5. "Near miss" answers typical
6. Patients highlight disabilities	6. Patients conceal disabilities
7. Patients often make little effort to perform well	7. Patients often struggle to perform well
8. Markedly variable performance on tasks of similar difficulty	8. Consistently poor performance on tasks of similar difficulty
9. Affective change often pervasive	9. Affect labile and shallow
10. Behavior often incongruent with manifested cognitive impairment	10. Behavior usually compatible with degree of cognitive loss

D. Among the more common treatable dementias that are referred to the psychiatrist in the emergency room are:

1. Pseudodementia—Dementia and depressive illness may be strikingly similar. Poor performance on mental status examination is frequently due to the inattention and apathy of depression. Apparent dementia on the basis of psychological impairment is called "pseudo-dementia." This condition can be a difficult diagnosis to make. Wells (1978b) has listed several differential diagnostic clues (Table III) which are helpful in distinguishing depression from dementia.

2. Wernicke-Korsakoff's—commonly seen in patients with history of alcohol abuse. The presence of ataxia, nystagmus, ophthalmoplegia, or peripheral neuropathy confirms the diagnosis.

3. Metabolic abnormalities—These most commonly occur in elderly patients with elevated BUN secondary to urinary tract infection.

4. Hyponatremia—found frequently in elderly patients on diuretics.

5. Drug or medication toxicity—over-the-counter medication or physician-prescribed medications.

6. Pneumonia—frequent in older patients and in alcoholics.

E. Treatment—The emergency room management of dementia is the same as delirium; however, the total treatment of dementia is generally beyond the scope of the emergency physician. It frequently involves medical, neurological, psychological and psychosocial intervention. The emergency physician is often the first professional person to come into contact with the patient. He will initiate the evaluation while others will provide the treatment. The emergency physician serves a vital function, because without his intervention many elderly patients will be diagnosed as senile dementia secondary to old age and sent home without the benefit of a comprehensive medical evaluation.

References

1. Alpers, B.J. and Mancall, E.L. *Essentials of the Neurological Examination,* F.A. Davis Company, Philadelphia, 1971.
2. Anderson, W. Emergency Department in *Handbook of General Hospital Psychiatry,* edited by Hackett and Caseem, C.V. Mosby Co., St. Louis, 1978, pp. 392–404.
3. Bannister, R. *Brains Clinical Neurology,* 4th edition. Oxford University Press, London, 1973.
4. Bellak, L. Enabling Conditions for the Ambulatory Psychotherapy of Acute Schizophrenics, Chapter 4 in *Specialized Techniques of Psychotherapy,* edited by T.B. Karasu and L. Bellak, Brunner/Mazel, New York, 1980.
5. Bellak, L. and Small, L. *Emergency Psychotherapy and Brief Psychotherapy,* 2nd edition, Grune and Stratton, New York, 1978.

6. Donlin, P., Hopkins, J., Tupin, J.D. Overview: Efficacy and Safety of Rapid Neuroleptization Method with Injectable Haldol. *American Journal of Psychiatry*, 136:273–278, 1979.

7. Dubin, W.R. and Zeccardi, J. "Medical Clearance of Organic Brain Syndrome in the Emergency Department: A Medical Dilemma," presented to the University Association of Emergency Medicine, Tuscon, AZ, April, 1980.

8. Biggs, J.T., Spiker, D.G., Petit, J.M., et al. Tricyclic Antidepressant Overdose, *JAMA*, 238:135–138, 1977.

9. London, W.P. Tips on Studying for the Psychiatry Boards. *Resident and Staff Physician,* October, 1978, pp. 119–123.

10. Morse, R.M. Psychiatry and Surgical Delirium, Chapter 30 in *Modern Perspective in the Psychiatric Aspects of Surgery,* edited by J.G. Howells, Brunner/Mazel, New York, 1976.

11. Murray, G.B. Confusion, Delirium and Dementia in *Handbook of General Hospital Psychiatry,* edited by Hackett and Cassem, C.V. Mosby Co., St. Louis, 1978, pp. 93–116.

12. *The Psychiatric Clinics of North America* V. 1, no. 1. Hugh C. Hendrie, editor, "Brain Disorders: Clinical Diagnosis and Management," W.B. Saunders Company, Philadelphia, 1978.

13. Seltzer, B. and Frazier, S.H. "Organic Mental Disorders," Chapter 15, in *The Harvard Guide to Modern Psychiatry,* edited by Armand M. Nicholi, Jr., Belknap Press of Harvard University Press, Cambridge, Mass., 1978, pp. 297–318.

14. Shevitz, S. Emergency Management of the Agitated Patient, *Primary Care,* Vol. 5, no. 4, pp. 625–634, 1978.

15. Slaby, A.E., Liev, J. and Tancredi, L.R. *Handbook of Psychiatric Emergencies,* 2nd edition. Medical Examination Publishing Co., Flushing, N.Y., 1980.

16. Weiner, H.L., Levitt, L.P. *Neurology for the House Officer,* 2nd edition, Williams and Wilkins Co., Baltimore, 1978.

17. Wells, Charles E. Chronic Brain Disease: An Overview. *American Journal of Psychiatry,* 135:1–12, 1978.

18. Wells, Charles E. Geriatric Organic Psychoses. *Psychiatric Annals,* 8:466–478, 1978b.

19. Wells, Charles E. and Duncan, Gary W. *Neurology for Psychiatrists.* F.A. Davis Co., Philadelphia, 1980.

20. *Psychiatric Presentations of Medical Illness,* edited by Richard C. Hall, M.D., SP Medical and Scientific Books, Jamaica, New York, 1980.

Chapter 4
Psychosis

Introduction

A. Psychotic patients frequently present in the emergency department out of control, manifesting bizarre behavior and speech, and are occasionally verbally abusive and physically threatening. Because they are often threatening, physicians will avoid psychotic patients or react in such a way as to inadvertently aggravate the patient's psychotic behavior. However, an understanding of psychosis can help the physician to develop a rational, meaningful treatment plan.

Psychotic disorders are characterized by varying degrees of personality disorganization. The patient may lose contact with reality or misperceive it to varying degrees. As a result, his capacity for effective work and interpersonal relations are impaired. Generally, psychosis results when there is an impairment of:

1. Mood—elation or depression
2. Thought, perception—schizophrenia
3. Orientation, memory, judgment and intellect—organic brain syndromes

There are several myths that exist about psychosis which frequently mislead physicians in the diagnosis and treatment of psychotic disorders. To avoid these mistakes it is helpful to remember that:

35

1. Delusions and hallucinations are not pathognomonic for schizophrenia and can occur in all types of psychotic disorders including mania, depression, and organic brain syndromes.

2. Differentiation of the psychotic illnesses is important since each illness has a specific pharmacological and psychotherapeutic treatment.

3. There are times when psychotic patients may not appear to be in contact with reality. However, part of their personality is usually intact and aware of what is happening, thus an obvious lack of respect and empathy for the patient's illness can seriously interfere with treatment.

Diagnosis

A. The diagnosis of schizophrenia is a much debated question in current psychiatry. There are many diagnostic approaches to the disease and no one approach has been demonstrated to be superior. Criteria used by the DSM-III is a middle-of-the-road diagnostic approach that incorporates the features of several different diagnostic systems. The DSM-III diagnostic schema not only takes into consideration the presence of symptoms during the acute phase, but also considers age of onset, duration, and course of the illness and previous level of functioning. The diagnostic criteria for schizophrenia according to DSM-III is as follows:

a) At least one of the following during a phase of the illness:
   1. bizarre delusions (content is patently absurd and has no possible basis in fact), such as delusions of being controlled, thought broadcasting, thought insertion, or thought withdrawal
   2. somatic, grandiose, religious, nihilistic, or other delusions without persecutory or jealous content
   3. delusions with persecutory or jealous content, if accompanied by hallucinations of any type
   4. auditory hallucinations in which either a voice keeps up a running commentary on the individual's behavior or thoughts, or two or more voices converse with each other
   5. auditory hallucinations on several occasions with content of

more than one or two words, having no apparent relation to either depression or elation

6. incoherence, marked loosening of associations, markedly illogical thinking, or marked poverty of content of speech, associated with at least one of the following:

- blunted, flat or inappropriate affect
- delusions or hallucinations
- catatonic or other grossly disorganized behavior

b) Deterioration from a previous level of functioning in such areas as work, social relations, and self care.

c) Duration: Continuous signs of the illness for at least six months at some time during the person's life, with some signs of the illness at present. The six-month period must include an active phase during which there were symptoms from (A), with or without a prodromal or residual phase, as defined below.

Prodromal phase: A clear deterioration in functioning before the active phase of the illness, not due to a disturbance in mood or to a substance use disorder and involving at least two of the symptoms noted below.

Residual phase: Persistence, following the active phase of the illness, of at least two of the symptoms noted below, not due to a disturbance in mood or to a substance use disorder.

Prodromal or Residual Symptoms:

1. social isolation or withdrawal
2. marked impairment in role-functioning as wage earner, student, or homemaker
3. markedly peculiar behavior (e.g., collecting garbage, talking to self in public, or hoarding food)
4. marked impairment in personal hygiene and grooming
5. blunted, flat, or inappropriate affect
6. digressive, vague, overelaborate, circumstantial or metaphorical speech
7. odd or bizarre ideation, or magical thinking, e.g., superstitiousness, clairvoyance, telepathy, "sixth sense," "others can feel my feelings," overvalued ideas, ideas of reference

8. unusual perceptual experiences, e.g., recurrent illusions, sensing the presence of a force or person not actually present.

d) Onset of prodromal or active phase of the illness before age 45.

e) Not due to any organic mental disorder or mental retardation.

Source: *Diagnostic and Statistical Manual of Mental Disorders: DSM-III*, Third Edition, American Psychiatric Association, 1980.

B. Manic-depressive psychosis—A major affective disorder characterized by severe mood swings and a tendency to remission and recurrence.

1. Manic type—consists of excessive elation, irritability, flight of ideas, talkativeness, motor hyperactivity, decreased sleep, shopping sprees and grandiosity. The patient may have grandiose or persecutory delusions. Auditory hallucinations may also be present. Manics can be very likable and amusing and maintain good rapport with the interviewer. Their interpersonal relationships and work history tend to be satisfactory between manic episodes. Frequently, there is a family history of affective disorder, alcoholism or sociopathy.

2. Depressed type—characterized by anhedonia, depressed mood, loss of appetite with weight loss, insomnia (especially early-morning awakening), psychomotor retardation, *or* agitation, somatic complaints, feelings of helplessness, hopelessness. Patients may have delusions of guilt, worthlessness or somatic delusions. Their work history and interpersonal relationships also tend to be satisfactory between depressive episodes.

C. Organic Brain Syndrome—characterized by impairment of cognitive functions (see Chapter 3).

D. Paranoid disorder—This disorder is characterized by persistent delusions of jealousy or persecution without any other evidence of schizophrenia, affective, or organic disorder. The onset is in late or middle life. Intellectual and occupational functioning remain intact while social and marital functioning are impaired. There are usually no hallucinations and the course is chronic.

E. Brief Reactive Psychosis—This disorder is characterized by a sudden onset following an immediate psychosocial stressor. The symptoms last from a couple of hours to less than 2 weeks with a return to the pre-morbid level of functioning. Symptoms include:

   a.   incoherence
   b.   delusions
   c.   hallucinations
   d.   disorganized or catatonic behavior

Treatment

A. In the acute phase, the management of psychosis is the same regardless of diagnosis. The goal of treatment in the emergency room is to alleviate the patient's tension; anxiety, confusion, and distress. If treatment intervention is successful, then in many instances hospitalization can be avoided and definitive treatment can be initiated in an outpatient clinic.

Even if hospitalization cannot be avoided, appropriate treatment will greatly reduce the risks of the patient harming himself or others and help establish a therapeutic rapport that will carry over in the in-patient setting and render the patient more compliant in his own treatment.

The clinical interview is the most important component of the emergency department treatment process. Not only does the interview serve as a means to gather data but also it is a therapeutic tool which can be used to provide support to the patient and gain his cooperation in the treatment process.

It is important to remember that psychosis is a *painful* experience. In spite of his psychosis, the patient is aware of what is happening to him and is frightened that he has no control over his behavior. A supportive empathic approach will help the patient to overcome his embarrassment and encourage him to participate in his treatment. The interviewer should remember that there is nothing mystical about psychosis. The interview should proceed in a systematic manner with the interviewer collecting the following data:

   1.   Present illness
   2.   Past medical and psychiatric history
   3.   Social history
   4.   Mental status
   5.   Physical examination

The interviewer should question the presence of delusions, hallucinations or other psychiatric symptomatology in a matter-of-fact manner. If a particular type of patient makes the interviewer extremely anxious or uncomfortable then the interviewer should consider asking someone else to interview the patient. The interviewer's uncontrolled anxiety may further agitate the patient.

Other useful techniques for interviewing psychotic patients are:

1. The interviewer should introduce himself, even if the patient seems confused. It is helpful to call the patient Mr. Smith rather than by his first name, e.g., Joe, etc.

2. The interview should begin with general, less intrusive questions, i.e., weather, work, school or any uncontroversial topic. As the rapport develops, the patient will feel more comfortable answering questions about the reasons that brought him to the emergency department.

3. The interviewer should avoid asking questions that can be answered yes or no. However, questions should be concise and direct, i.e., "Tell me what happened?"

4. The interviewer must actively assist the patient in defining problems and focusing on issues. When the interviewer has difficulty understanding the patient, he should be supportive of the patient. Rather than berating him, i.e., "You're not making any sense," the interviewer could say, "I'm having difficulty following you." "Do you mean. . .," or "Would you repeat that again?"

5. When interest in the patient's history is displayed, this frequently contributes to a positive relationship in which the patient perceives that he will receive help, and as a result his agitation and anxiety will be further attenuated.

B. If a patient's anxiety or agitation is interfering with or preventing the interview, then tranquilization without sedation, using neuroleptics, should be attempted. Tablets have a long absorption time and therefore they are not helpful in the acute treatment. Intramuscular medication or concentrate form are much more rapidly absorbed and equally effective. The majority of patients will comply and take the concentrate in orange juice. This form is much more palatable to the patient than intramuscular injection. The dosage range is as follows:

Drug	Dose (concentrate or I.M.)
Navane (Thiothixene)	10–15 mg q 30 minutes
Stelazine (Trifluoperazine)	10–15 mg q 30 minutes
Haldol (Haloperidol)	5–10 mg q 30 minutes
Serentil (Mesoridazine)	25 mg q 30 minutes sedating drugs
Thorazine (Chlorpromazine)	25–50 mg q 30 minutes sedating drugs
Mellaril (Thioridazine)	25–50 mg q 30 minutes sedating drugs

The doses should be repeated until tranquilization is achieved, usually 1 to 3 doses will effectively tranquilize the patient. Rapid tranquilization should be used to reduce the patient's anxiety, agitation, tension, confusion, and belligerence. It is important to remember that hallucinations and delusions will persist since these symptoms require 1-6 weeks of neuroleptic treatment before remission occurs. Although these doses are not of equivalent potency, empirical use suggests that these doses produce the most satisfactory results.

C. It is useful to remember that:

1. Serentil, Mellaril and Thorazine are the most sedating drugs and should be used when a patient is so agitated that sedation is desired. The need for these drugs occurs most frequently with manic patients.

2. Navane and Haldol have the weakest anticholinergic actions and are preferable for elderly patients, patients with hypotensive problems or cardiac problems.

3. These drugs have a wide margin of safety and high doses can be achieved rapidly.

4. Blood pressure should be taken prior to every dose. A systolic pressure of <100 and a diastolic of <60 is an indication to withhold medication until the blood pressure returns to normal.

When the physician determines that the patient requires medication, he should offer the medication in a firm, direct manner, i.e., "I can see that you are upset (or nervous) and I would like to give you some medicine to help you relax." Most patients will comply with this request since they want relief from their symptoms. Tricking the patient by slipping medication into water or juice is a desperate ploy that should be avoided. Patients fear being "put to sleep" by neuroleptic medication and it is helpful to reassure them that the medicine will help them feel more relaxed and not put them to sleep.

After the acute phase of evaluation and treatment has been accomplished, the physician can determine the most appropriate disposition. Some guidelines for disposition include:

1. Admit to hospital if patient shows no improvement with medication and interview.

2. Admit if patient improves, but remains so psychotic that he is unable to care for his daily needs, i.e., economic, housing, grooming, etc.

3. Admit if patient is psychotic and poses a physical threat to himself or others.

4. Admit if it is the first psychotic episode for the patient.

5. Admit if patient is having command hallucinations, i.e., voices telling him to act in a destructive manner.

6. Admit if in doubt about severity of condition.

7. Discharge if patient improves with medication and supportive therapy and has supportive environment to return to.

8. Discharge if patient improves with medication and supportive therapy and has long history (10 years or more) of psychotic functioning without any appreciable change over this period of time. Many of these patients come to the emergency department seeking food and shelter.

If patient is unemployed, does not attend school, and tends to spend most of his time withdrawn, or if a patient works part-time but has few social supports, referral to a Partial Hospital Program is preferable. If a patient is working or attends school and has a supportive system, out-patient treatment will usually suffice.

References

1. Anderson, W.H. The Emergency Department, in *Massachusetts General Hospital Handbook of General Hospital Psychiatry*, edited by Thomas P. Hackett and Ned H. Cassem. The C.V. Mosby Co., St. Louis, 1978, pp. 392–404.
2. Appleton, W.S. and Davis, J.M. *Practical Clinical Psychopharmacology*, 2nd edition, Williams and Wilkins, Baltimore, 1980.
3. Bellak, L. and Small, L. *Emergency Psychotherapy and Brief Psychotherapy*, 2nd edition. Grune and Stratton, New York, 1967.
4. *Diagnostic and Statistical Manual of Mental Disorders: DSM-III*, Third Edition, American Psychiatric Association, Division of Public Affairs, 1700 18th Street, N.W., Washington, D.C., 1980.
5. Donlon, P.T., Hopkin, J. and Tupin, J.P. Overview: Efficacy and Safety of the Rapid Neuroleptization Method with Injectable Haloperidol. *American Journal of Psychiatry*, 136:273–278, 1978.
6. Ketai, R. Psychotropic Drugs in the Management of Psychiatric Emergencies, *Postgraduate Medicine*, 58:87–93, 1975.
7. Klerman, G.L. Affective Disorders, Chapter 13, in *The Harvard Guide to Modern Psychiatry*, Armand M. Nicholi, Jr., editor, Belknap Press of Harvard University Press, Cambridge, Mass., 1978, pp. 253–279.
8. MacKinnon, R.A. and Michels, R. *The Psychiatric Interview in Clinical Practice*. W.B. Saunders Company, Philadelphia, 1971.
9. Stotsky, B.A. Relative Efficacy of Parenteral Haloperidol and Thiothixene for the Emergency Treatment of Acutely Excited and Agitated Patients. *Diseases of the Nervous System*, 38:967–973, 1977.
10. Strauss, J.S. The Treatment of Outpatient Schizophrenics. *The Journal of Continuing Education in Psychiatry*, 38:23–34, 1977.
11. Strauss, J.S. and Gift, T.E. Choosing an Approach for Diagnosing Schizophrenia. *Archives of General Psychiatry*, v. 34, October 1977, pp. 1248–1253.
12. Taylor, M.A. and Abrams, R. The Phenomenology of Mania. *Archives of General Psychiatry*, 29:520–522, 1973.

Chapter 5
Non-Psychotic Disturbances

Introduction

Patients often present to the emergency department because of psychological problems which have been unresolved and have resulted in psychiatric and/or physical symptoms. Though the patient is not psychotic, he is in distress. Usually he has little if any insight into the psychological dynamics of his discomfort and comes to the emergency department seeking relief from his symptoms. The patients with anxiety disorders and grief reactions fall into this group of patients.

A. Anxiety Disorders

Patients that present to the emergency department with anxiety are usually in a state of panic which has resulted from an environmental stress or from instinctual impulses that the patient fears he can no longer control, e.g., aggression or sexual feelings, fears of passivity, etc. Extreme anxiety is indicative of heightened tension and reflects the inability of the patient's psychological defense mechanisms to master the stress. When the patient is seen in the emergency department, he is usually helpless, out of control, and fearful of complete personality disintegration. The presenting symptoms are predominantly physical and include:

1. tachycardia
2. palpitations

3. extrasystoles
4. restlessness
5. sense of air hunger
6. sweating
7. dizziness
8. light-headedness
9. fine tremor
10. heartburn
11. G.I. distress
12. musculo-skeletal aches and pains
13. hyperventilation
14. a feeling of impending doom
15. fears of becoming insane
16. fears of becoming violent

Differential Diagnosis—though a psychological etiology is the precipitating cause for a large percentage of anxiety disorders, an emergency department evaluation must also include a consideration of physical causes. These include:

1. Caffeinism
2. Cerebral hypoxia—secondary to cardiac or pulmonary abnormalities
3. Cushing's disease
4. Alcohol or sedative withdrawal
5. Amphetamines
6. Steroids
7. Hyperthyroidism
8. Hypoglycemia

The list of these 8 conditions is summarized in the mnemonic, "$C_3A_2S\ H_2$" (London, 1978).

Treatment

The goal of treating the patient with anxiety in the emergency room is to establish an emotional equilibrium for the patient and help him regain mastery over his thoughts and feelings. At the point of intervention in the emergency room there is no attempt to bring about characterological change and insight therapy is generally of limited value. Treatment guidelines are as follows:

1. Since the patient feels helpless and frightened, a direct approach will help to alleviate the patient's symptoms. The patient should be given reassurance that his problems are controllable and that he can be helped. The patient should be given a direct explanation of his symptoms and his unrealistic fears should be pointed out, e.g., explain that his tachycardia does not mean he is having a heart attack. It is helpful to reassure him that he is not going insane.

2. The patient should be encouraged to express his feelings and thoughts. Not only will this help establish a rapport with the interviewer but it will also provide the patient with an outlet for his tension.

3. By pointing out to the patient other areas in his life in which he has been successful, the interviewer will increase the patient's feeling of competence and help him to realize that he is not as helpless as he thought.

4. Other therapeutic interventions might include providing guidance for the patient. Patients who are paralyzed by their anxiety may require suggestions as to how to organize their time, in order to prevent them from sitting around ruminating about their problem. At times, environmental manipulation may be necessary, e.g., suggesting that the patient live with family or friends a few days, not go to work for several days or continue to work, etc. Mobilizing the support of friends and family may be helpful with some patients. At times it is helpful to interview family members and/or friends since they can frequently provide a more comprehensive history than a highly anxious patient. The family's presence may help to increase the patient's feeling of being supported and cared for.

5. When a patient is seen in the emergency department, his anxiety is often so intense that it can interfere with efforts to interview and treat him. Minor tranquilizers are useful in these cases and one or two doses will serve to attenuate the anxiety.

Drugs that may be used include:

Librium (chlordiazepoxide)	10–25 mg, p.o.
Valium (diazepam)	5–10 mg, p.o.
Ativan (lorazepam)	1–2 mg, p.o.
Serax (oxazepam)	15–30 mg, p.o.

These can be given twice or three times a day for 2 or 3 days after discharge from the emergency room. Neuroleptics should not be used initially to treat anxiety disorders unless the anxiety is secondary to a psychotic process.

6. When the patient is discharged, the interviewer should arrange an outpatient appointment since further evaluation and therapy will usually be necessary to help the patient understand the underlying psychological issues which resulted in the anxiety attack. Without therapy the patient is at risk of future relapses. The appointment should be made as soon as possible, because a patient who finds relief from the emergency intervention will feel less inclined to follow up as an outpatient if he remains asymptomatic after discharge. The patient should be reassured that he can contact the physician at any time.

B. Grief Reaction

The grief reaction represents the conscious impact of a loss to an individual. The loss may be a result of a death or the loss of a body part, e.g., amputation or an economic loss such as a job. Uncomplicated grief is a normal response to loss and generally runs a benign course. However, when the normal grieving process does not occur, patients may present in the emergency department with a pathological grief reaction which can manifest as depression, alcoholism, phobia, anxiety attacks and severe disruptions of their personal life, e.g., marriage, work, schooling. When patients present with a secondary psychiatric problem, the interviewer can establish that a pathological grief reaction is occurring by eliciting a significant loss in the patient's life and/or establishing the presence of the symptoms of grief. These symptoms include:

1. Somatic distress which is manifested by feelings of fatigue, sighing respirations, shortness of breath, dizziness, blurred vision, palpitations, frequent ongoing episodes and feelings of numbness.

2. Preoccupation with the image of the deceased to such a degree that the patient may actually think he sees or hears the deceased.

3. Preoccupation with guilt feelings in which the patient feels that perhaps he contributed in some way to the loss or feels guilty of his past negligence toward the deceased.

4. Feelings of hostility which are frequently directed toward the hospital staff for not properly caring for the deceased. Frequently a more covert theme is hostility toward the deceased for abandoning the patient. The hostility can be manifested by the patient complaining of a loss of the warm, tender feelings that he had toward other family members and friends.

5. A disruption of normal life patterns such as sleep, appetite, work, or normal relations with other people.

One situation in which the emergency room physician can be helpful in facilitating a normal grief reaction is when there is a sudden unexpected death. This can occur with the death of a patient after arrival at the hospital, stillbirth, sudden infant death, accidental or traumatic death, cardiac arrest, death during or after surgery, murder or suicide.

Treatment

Each patient reacts differently to grief. The reaction is not only influenced by personality style, but also by cultural mores. The initial evaluation of the patient must include an assessment of the degree of depression, the presence or absence of psychosis, alcoholism and suicidal potential. If hospitalization is not necessary, then treatment can begin in the emergency room.

1. The patient should be encouraged to talk about his feelings and thoughts concerning the deceased. The interviewer should question the patient in a way that will encourage the patient to begin reviewing his past relationship with the deceased.

2. Reassure the patient that symptoms such as preoccupation with images of the deceased, insomnia, somatic distress, and social withdrawal are normal reactions in grief and that by discussing his

feelings and thoughts these symptoms will gradually attenuate. The patient should be reassured that he is not losing his mind.

3. If feelings of hostility and anger are overt, the patient should be encouraged to discuss these feelings. Angry feelings toward hospital staff for not preventing the loss should be viewed in the context of the grief reaction and not be personalized by the interviewer. If the patient alludes to angry feelings toward the deceased, then the interviewer should encourage the patient to discuss these feelings.

4. The patient should be encouraged to establish new relationships. All efforts should be made to have the patient return to his past activities such as work and school. Frequently it is helpful to mobilize family and friends by having them come into the emergency room and explaining to them that the patient's symptoms are part of a grief reaction. This knowledge will often unify family and friends into a more supportive role.

5. When a sudden unexpected death occurs, management of the patient is generally similar to that of the grief reaction. Questions which help the patient review the last memories of the deceased will help begin the normal grieving process. It is important to allow the grieving process to begin and no attempt should be made to stop the process with sedation or statements such as "it's God's will."

6. Because personnel in the emergency room usually have no established relationship with the patient, it is helpful to notify family and/or friends and encourage them to come to the emergency department, since they can help provide support for the patient.

7. Patients cope with loss differently. Some patients will ventilate freely and with frequent emotional outbursts. Other patients, however, are quiet and reserved with little overt expression of any feelings. The physician should not assume that quiet patients are "handling the situation" and then leave them alone. The physician can provide comfort for these patients by just sitting with them. The silence can be a reflection of the shock that the patient feels and the quiet presence of staff keeps open the possibility of ventilation as the patient's numbness diminishes.

8. The patient and/or family should be offered a chance to view the body. If the body is mutilated the family should be warned that the body is disfigured; however, if they insist on seeing the victim then they should be allowed to do so.

9. In all grief reactions, sedation should be used sparingly. If the patient, however, requires some tranquilization, then a minor tranquilizer such as Valium 5-10 mg, Librium 10-25 mg, Ativan 1-2 mg or Serax 15-30 mg may be used. The medication should be used to reduce the anxiety level, and sedation should be avoided.

10. When the patient is discharged, he should be given an outpatient appointment as soon as possible and should be reassured that he can contact the physician if needed. The patients, when possible, should be accompanied home by family or friends and should not spend the night by themselves. Patients who have experienced a sudden unexpected loss should be made aware of the availability of outpatient and emergency services should they feel a need to talk further with a professional.

Personality Disorders

These are patients who have developed a maladaptive pattern of responding to social, occupational, or psychological distress. When overwhelmed by environmental or psychological stresses, they will frequently come to the emergency department with the hope that the treating personnel will help them solve their current problems. Among the most frequent personality disorders seen in the emergency room are the borderline, the histrionic and the antisocial personalities.

A. Borderline Personality

There are six characteristics of the borderline personality that can be helpful in its diagnosis. They include:

1. Psychotic episodes that are usually brief and paranoid in nature.

2. Psychological test performance that is poorer on unstructured

tests such as the Rorschach, but better on structured tests such as the Wechsler Adult Intelligence Scale.

3. A history of impulsive behavior such as drug and alcohol abuse, self-mutilation, suicidal gestures, promiscuity, gambling, shoplifting, bulimia.

4. Interpersonal relationships that are usually unstable, transient, superficial, or intensely dependent. Relationships are characterized by the consistent use of others to meet their own ends.

5. Affect that is intense, angry with lack of control of anger. There can be frequent shifts from normal mood to depression.

6. Adaptiveness to social situations is not impaired (achievement in school or work, appropriate appearance, social awareness). These symptoms can be remembered by the mnemonic $(PIA)^2$.

Treatment

a) Because of the wide range of presenting symptoms, borderline personalities can fall into almost any category of emergency psychiatry, i.e., psychosis, violence, suicide, drug and alcohol, and transient situational disturbances. In treating these patients, the physician must first determine which problem requires immediate attention and treat according to the guidelines given for each of these conditions in the appropriate chapter.

b) If hospitalization is not required, the physician can initiate treatment in the emergency department. However, one must be reminded that borderline patients can be difficult to treat because of the myriad of feelings that they arouse in therapists. These feelings range from apathy to rage.

c) The borderline patient with interpersonal difficulties will tend to blame someone else and present in the emergency room with the expectation that the physician can manipulate the environment on his behalf. Rather than interpret this or become angry at the manipulative attempt, the physician should explore the events that precipitated the emergency.

d) Frequently with borderline patients, limits and structure have to be set. The patient must be told at times what behavior is unacceptable in the emergency department, e.g., violence, verbal abuse, etc. This should be done with a firm, concise explanation avoiding expression of impatience or anger.

e) The patient should be allowed to ventilate feelings. This frequently takes time and the physician cannot be too impatient.

f) Minor tranquilizers or low-dose neuroleptic medication can further help to alleviate the patient's anxiety when necessary.

B. Histrionic Personality

The histrionic personality has a history of behavior patterns characterized by excitability, emotional instability, over-reactivity, and self-dramatization. This self-dramatization is always attention-seeking and often seductive, whether or not the patient is aware of its purpose. These personalities are also immature, self-centered, often vain, and usually dependent on others. These patients are frequently seen in the emergency department after interpersonal disappointment.

Treatment

a) The physician should be aware of the patient's anxiety and readiness for emotional overinvolvement, and should proceed with a measure of calmness and firmness to avoid stirring up these reactions. Do not try to calm the patient with rationalizations.

b) Because histrionic patients tend to be dependent they will attempt to have the physician assume responsibility for their decisions. The physician should empathize with the patient's problems *but* should encourage them to make their own decision; e.g., "Doctor, you're the first person who has really listened to me and seems to understand my problems. What do you think I should do? I know you will make the right decision for me."

The most helpful reply would be, "Up to now you have been able to manage this situation in spite of all the difficulties. What would you do next?"

c) Do not rush the disposition of the patient. This may cause an exacerbation of anxiety. Remember, these patients are in pain and have little insight into their problems. Give the patient ample time to ventilate.

d) If marked anxiety is a prevalent symptom, a single dose of a minor tranquilizer will frequently alleviate the symptoms and gratify the patient's need to be taken care of.

e) If the patient presents with suicidal gestures or threats, he should be managed according to the guidelines in Chapter 8.

f) The patients should know that after discharge they can contact the emergency department at any time for further help.

C. Antisocial Personality

These patients generally are seen in the emergency room with drug, alcohol, housing, or monetary problems. They generally will try to manipulate the hospital staff into manipulating other systems for them, e.g., welfare, social service, etc. When frustrated, they often pose a threat of violence.

Diagnostic criteria include:

a) A history of school problems, delinquency, alcohol or drug abuse and legal difficulties, all prior to age 15.

b) After age 15, poor work history, repeated legal problems, poor marital history, repeated physical fights, no sense of financial responsibility, failure to plan ahead, disregard for the truth and a history of impulsiveness.

Treatment

a) Remember, these patients may become violent when frustrated. With aggressive patients it is helpful to have security present and visible to the patient. Strict limits should be set without arguing or negotiating with the patient. If alcohol or drug problems are involved these should be evaluated according to the guidelines in Chapters 8 and 9. If the patient is agitated he may require medication. The safest management of these patients should follow the guidelines of the management of the violent patient (Chapter 7). When appropriate, social agencies can be contacted for help with housing, referral for welfare, etc. The patient should be referred to a Partial Hospital program when one is available.

There are other categories of patients that also fall into the non-psychotic group.

a) Intermittent explosive disorder—These are patients with a history of discrete episodes of loss of control with behavior that is out of proportion to any precipitating cause. These patients should be managed according to the guidelines in Chapter 7.

b) Hysterical Conversion Disorder is the loss or alteration of physical functioning that cannot be explained on a medical basis and is an expression of a psychological conflict. Generally, the workup, neurological and medical, is extensive since all possible physical etiologies should be considered. First episodes should be admitted for a complete medical and psychiatric evaluation. Patients that are known to have had previous episodes should be treated by psychiatrists. Treatment in the emergency department includes supportive therapy, persuasion, medication and/or placebos, family or marital intervention, and behavioral therapy. Frequently, the intervention required is so extensive that hospitalization is required in a psychiatric unit.

c) Adjustment Disorders—These disorders result from an identifiable psychosocial stressor that leads to an impairment of social or occupational functioning and results in symptoms that are in excess of what would be expected. The reaction usually occurs within three months of the onset of the stressor. Precipitants of adjustment reactions include accident, death, medical illness, divorce, job loss, mugging, rape or abortion, etc. Symptoms can include anxious or depressed mood, impaired school or academic performance, and emotional withdrawal. The emergency room treatment is the same as treatment of the anxiety disorders. After discharge, the patient should be referred for out-patient therapy.

References

1. Bellak, L. and Small, L. *Emergency Psychotherapy and Brief Psychotherapy,* 2nd edition. Grune and Stratton, New York, 1967.
2. Cassem, N.H. Treating the Person Confronting Death, in *The Harvard Guide to Modern Psychiatry,* edited by A.M. Nicholi. Belknap Press of Harvard University Press, Cambridge, Mass., 1978, pp. 579–606.
3. *Diagnostic and Statistical Manual of Mental Disorders III,* American Psychiatric Association, Washington, D.C., 1980.
4. Lesse, S. Psychotherapy of Ambulatory Patients with Severe Anxiety, Chapter II, in *Specialized Techniques in Individual Psychotherapy,* edited by T.B. Karasu and L. Bellak, Brunner/Mazel, New York, 1980.
5. London, W.P. Tips on Studying for the Psychiatry Boards. *Resident and Staff Physician,* October 1978, pp. 119–123.
6. Nemiah, J.C. Psychoneurotic Disorders, in *The Harvard Guide to Modern Psychiatry,* edited by A.M. Nicholi. Belknap Press of Harvard University Press, Cambridge, Mass., 1978, pp. 173–197.
7. Pfeiffer, E. Borderline States. *Diseases of the Nervous System,* 35: 212–219, 1974.
8. Shapiro, E. Psychodynamics and Developmental Psychology of the Borderline Patient: A Review of the Literature. *American Journal of Psychiatry,* 135:1304–1315, 1978.
9. Wolberg, L.R. *The Technique of Psychotherapy, Parts 1 and 2,* 2nd edition, Grune and Stratton, New York, 1967.

Chapter 6

The Violent Patient

Introduction

Most physicians in emergency departments will avoid violent patients because intervention frequently results in verbal abuse and physical threats. Furthermore, the patients are non-compliant and are generally brought in by family and police for treatment against their will. Mismanagement of the violent patient can result in physical harm to emergency room staff and destruction of property. The most effective management for the violent patient is preventive management, and this prevention depends on *early recognition* of signals of potential violence and a response that will defuse the threat.

Prediction of Violence—Diagnostic Clues

The earliest clues as to the potential violence of a patient are based on diagnosis. Certain diagnostic groups which seem to have a higher propensity for violence include:

A. *Drug intoxications*—Patients who are intoxicated from alcohol or drugs, especially amphetamine, LSD or phencyclidine (angel dust), have a much greater potential for violence.

B. *Drug or alcohol withdrawals*—Patients in withdrawal often attempt to manipulate staff for more drugs to ward off their withdrawal and when they are refused drugs by medical personnel they often become very threatening and abusive. Patients in delirium tremens can be extremely violent.

C. *Acute organic brain syndromes* (delirium)—The potential for violence in these patients is often not appreciated by the medical staff who often become preoccupied with the medical problem of the patient. Conversely the presenting symptom of patients with delirium is frequently agitated, combative behavior.

D. *Post-ictal state*—Violence usually occurs when the patient presents in the emergency department in a post-ictal state and staff fails to recognize that the patient has had a seizure.

E. *Acute psychosis*—This includes patients with acute schizophrenic episodes and patients that are acutely manic. Manic patients are more dangerous because staff gain a false sense of security with the manic's expansive mood and good humor. Manics, however, can become quite violent when limits are placed on them.

F. *Paranoid personality*—Paranoid personalities pose a potential for violence especially when the examiner begins a probing interview despite the patient's resistance and warning to the physician to leave him alone.

G. *Antisocial and borderline personalities*—Frequently violent when they present with drug and alcohol withdrawal or intoxications.

H. Other diagnostic categories that are frequently cited as being potentially violent include temporal lobe epilepsy and pathological intoxication.

Behavioral Clues

The most important predictors of potential violence are the patient's *behavioral clues* (Hackett, 1977), which include:

A. *Posture* —Observe how the patient is sitting during the interview. Is the patient comfortable or relaxed? If the patient is *sitting on the edge of the chair or gripping the armrests,* the interviewer should be cautious and alerted to the potential for violence. The greater the tension in the posture, the greater the risk of violence.

B. *Speech* —How is the patient talking during the interview? Is he talking in a calm voice, or is his *voice loud and strident?* Does the patient seem to get louder and louder as the interview goes on? The *louder and more strident,* the greater the potential for violence, especially if the interviewer overreacts to the verbal stridency.

C. *Motor activity* —The most important and most ignored sign of impending violence is the patient's motor activity. Patients who are anxious and restless and keep pacing around the examining room or in the halls pose the most serious threat of violence. *This behavior is considered a psychiatric emergency which demands immediate intervention.*

D. *Startle response* —If the patient startles easily this could be a sign of impending drug or alcohol withdrawal.

The most important data from the patient's past history that is helpful in predicting violence is a past history of violence. If the patient has a history of impulsive violence when his needs are frustrated or not satisfied, then the patient is a much higher risk for violence.

If the patient falls into the pertinent diagnostic categories, has a past history of violence, and the behavioral clues are present, then immediate intervention is necessary.

Management of the Violent Patient

A. Proper management of violent patients follows a logical progression of therapeutic interventions beginning with:

1. *Talk* —Ask the patient in a direct, firm manner "How can we help you?" Most patients appreciate that someone bothers to ask what is going on and very frequently will feel great relief that they have

someone to talk with. Begin the interview with benign topics, e.g., job, schooling, weather, etc. Only after the patient shows some degree of relaxation and rapport with the examiner is the present illness discussed. If the patient is loud, talk softly. He will often lower his voice so he can hear. Loud profane speech should be regarded as a symptom, and the interviewer should avoid getting into a shouting contest with the patient. The technique of talking to a psychotic patient (Chapter 4) is also valid and useful in talking to a violent patient.

2. *Food* — If talking does not defuse the situation then offer the patient something to eat or drink. Food has a calming effect on the patient's tension and anxiety and the physician is viewed as sincerely concerned about the patient when he offers food or drink. A helpful technique is to offer the patient coffee or juice at the time of introduction, e.g., "Hello, I'm Dr. Dubin. Would you like some coffee or juice?"

3. *Medication* — Tell the patient you can see he is upset and nervous and some medication will calm him down. In patients who are paranoid and reluctant to talk to the interviewer, the physician can tell the patient that he knows that he is having thoughts and feelings that are upsetting. He can suggest that some medication will help him feel more relaxed. Drug concentrates in orange juice are much more acceptable to patients than intramuscular medication. Avoid pills and capsules since the absorption takes too long to exert immediate effect. Effective doses are:

Drug	Dose (given q 30 minutes concentrate or I.M.)	
Navane	10–15 mg	
Stelazine	10–15 mg	
Haldol	5–10 mg	
Serentil	25 mg	
Mellaril	25–50 mg	more
Thorazine	25–50 mg	sedating

The dose can be repeated at 30-minute intervals until there is a reduction in the anxiety, tension and agitation that the patient is experiencing. However, it is important to remember that rapid tranquilization will not cause remission of hallucinations and delusions. This takes 1–6 weeks of appropriate neuroleptic treatment. As a rule, one to three doses is sufficient to induce tranquilization without sedation. If for some reason the patient cannot take neuroleptic medication then sodium amytal 250 mg intramuscularly can be used. Try to avoid sedation so that the patient can be interviewed.

4. *Support* – Utilize anyone in the emergency room who seems to have had some positive interaction with the patient. This might be a security guard, a family member, or a secretary. Have this person talk with the patient, under the direction of staff. Once the patient is calm, this person should attempt to persuade the patient to take some medication.

5. *Security guards* – If it is necessary to call the security guards use a code name in order to avoid inciting the patient. When security arrives, do not immediately rush into the patient's room. Instead, place the guards in positions where the patient can see them. Frequently their presence will reassure the patient that if he gets out of control there are enough personnel to restrain him. It is important for psychotic patients to feel that they will be prevented from losing control and harming themselves or others. A show of force is especially helpful with belligerent and threatening character disorders.

6. *Restraints* – The triad of (1) an agitated patient (2) with whom the physician cannot establish rapport and (3) who does not comply with the request to take medication or sit down, etc. and whose agitation does not subside or continues to increase, indicates that the patient should be placed in restraints. Once the decision is made to restrain the patient it should immediately be acted on. Negotiating with the patient is generally futile. When a patient is to be restrained staff should leave the room so that the security force can restrain the patient. A minimum of four people are necessary, one for each limb. Remember, patients *can also bite*. The presence of a nurse talking to the patient

while the security guards restrain him often calms him and renders the patient more compliant. Restraining a patient is a psychiatric emergency and all effort should be directed at getting the patient out of restraints. This usually involves rapid tranquilization and supportive therapy with the patient. Once in restraints, a patient should never be left unobserved.

Reversal of the above triad is a good indication that a patient can be let out of restraints. It is helpful to have security present when the patient is initially taken out of restraints.

B. There are several other helpful strategies in dealing with violent patients in addition to those outlined above. All patients should be evaluated with the interviewer between the patient and the door. Sitting behind a desk traps the interviewer. If the interviewer has any concern that the patient will become violent, then the interviewer should leave the door open during the interview and consider having additional personnel sit in on the interview. An effort should be made to avoid excessive stimulation, such as being near a loud patient, or being in a busy area. In agitated patients or paranoid personalities, the interviewer should stay at least arm's length away from the patient. Finally, staff should never turn their backs on a patient until a distance of 15 to 20 feet separate staff and patient.

If a patient has a weapon, the interviewer has the right to refuse to examine the patient until he either surrenders the weapon or allows security guards to search the patient and remove the weapon. If the patient will not surrender the weapon, the interviewer *should never* take the weapon from the patient but should have the patient place the weapon on the table or the floor; the interviewer can remove the weapon after the interview. The patient might instinctively pull the trigger if the interviewer approaches him. Finally, if a patient causes the interviewer to feel unduly anxious, the interviewer should ask someone else to interview the patient. *An interviewer who is out of control will only further increase the anxiety and agitation of the patient.*

References

1. Cohen, Sidney. Aggression: The Rule of Drugs, *Drug Abuse and Alcoholism Newsletter*, Vista Hill Foundation, Volume 8, No. 2, February, 1979.
2. DiBella, G.A.W. Educating Staff to Manage Threatening Paranoid Patients. *American Journal of Psychiatry*, 136:333–335, 1979.
3. Hackett, T. "The Management of the Violent Patient," presentation, Harvard Course in Emergency Psychiatry, July, 1977.
4. Lion, J.R. *Evaluation and Management of the Violent Patient*, Charles C. Thomas, Springfield, Illinois, 1972.
5. Rockwell, D.A. Can You Spot Potential Violence in a Patient? *Hospital Physician*, 10:52–56, 1972.

Chapter 7
The Suicidal Patient

Introduction

One of the true psychiatric emergencies occurs when a patient is suicidal. The suicidal patient should always be evaluated by a psychiatrist; however, there are times when no psychiatrist is immediately available, and some decision must be made as to the potential suicide risk of the patient. Generally, there are three types of patients that will present to the emergency room as suicide risks:

A. The first type will present with a chief complaint of suicidal thoughts without any overt gesture.

B. The second and most common type of patient presents with a suicide gesture in which he has not intended to kill himself but is acting in such a way as to attract attention or to "get back at someone." There is a tendency for physicians to take these patients lightly. However, these patients frequently will make another gesture and may kill themselves by mistake.

C. The third type of suicide attempt is made by patients with true suicidal intent who were saved only by unusual intervention.

Assessing the Suicidal Risk

A. Suicide attempts may occur across all diagnostic categories including neurosis, character disorders, psychosis, situational crises, organic brain syndromes and often in "normal" patients suffering from medical illnesses. In interviewing any patient, the examining physician should always ask if the patient has feelings or thoughts of killing himself. It is a myth to feel that the examining physician will give the patient the idea of suicide. If the patient wants to kill himself, he will have thought about it before the physician asks. If the patient answers "yes" to this question, then the physician should inquire further about the type of plan the patient has about committing suicide. If the patient comes into the emergency room with a suicide attempt, or gesture, then the physician must first make some assessment as to how serious the attempt was and whether the patient should be admitted to an inpatient unit, or can be treated in an outpatient clinic.

B. There are several criteria that are helpful for assessing suicide risk, but it must be stated that no method for assessing suicide potential is perfect. In the long run, one must weigh all the indices for and against a possible suicide attempt in order to assess the degree of seriousness. Helpful indices include:

1. *Seriousness of the suicide attempt:* the more lethal the attempt, the greater the suicide risk. A patient who cuts his wrist or attempts to hang or shoot himself is a more severe suicide risk than someone who has taken an overdose of 10 aspirin. However, the larger the overdose, the more serious the risk.

2. *Imminence of rescue:* when the patient plans the suicide so that rescue would be inevitable, the suicide risk is reduced; i.e., as soon as he took the pills, did the patient call a relative, or did he wait until everyone had left for the evening, and then attempt to shoot himself? The less imminent the chance of rescue, the greater the threat of suicide.

3. *Family and personal history:* if the patient has a past history of suicide attempts, or a family history of suicide attempts, the risk of suicide increases.

4. *Mental Status:* if the patient is psychotic, intoxicated by alcohol or drugs, the threat of suicide is increased.

C. In general, the risk of suicide is much higher in:

1. Older, single, divorced, or widowed males
2. Caucasians
3. Protestants
4. Unemployed patients
5. Patients in poor physical health
6. Patients that leave suicide notes
7. Patients living alone
8. Patients with an anniversary death or loss
9. Patients with sudden changes in life situation

Treatment

A. The suicide patient represents a true psychiatric emergency and no suicidal patient should be allowed to leave the emergency room without a psychiatric evaluation. The therapy of suicidal patients is generally diverse and should be left, in the main, to psychiatrists. However, there are times when a psychiatrist is not readily available and a non-psychiatrist must initiate treatment. In approaching the suicidal patient the physician should be objective, nonjudgmental, and concerned. Physicians should avoid the tactic of reprimanding patients for the suicide attempt but instead should attempt to focus on other positive areas of the patient's life accomplishments. It is also important to remember that the interview itself often provides the patient with an opportunity to discuss many of his feelings. Often, this ventilation of feelings will greatly diminish the suicide impulse. When evaluating the suicidal patient, it is recommended that:

1. Questions concerning suicide should be initially asked in the context of a general inquiry about feelings of depression and hopelessness, i.e., "How bad do you feel?" "What do you feel the future holds in store for you?" "If you have felt this bad before, can you describe what was happening?"

2. The examiner should specifically question the patient about his suicide plan. The interviewer can then determine the imminence of danger, i.e., someone who has vague thoughts of shooting himself is not quite as serious a risk as someone who is thinking of shooting himself and has a loaded gun at home.

3. The events and feelings of the patient prior to the patient's presenting to the emergency room should be established. By encouraging the patient to discuss his feelings and fantasies of suicide, the mystique of suicide is frequently debunked and the patient will begin to consider other alternatives.

4. The examining physician should also be aware of non-verbal communication, i.e., a patient who comes to the emergency room with his bags packed and is expecting to be admitted. Patients who recently made a will or straightened out financial affairs may not be expecting to live long.

B. If the patient is in treatment, the therapist should be notified of the suicidal gesture/attempt. Frequently the therapist can provide information that will facilitate the emergency treatment of the patient.

C. In certain cases, especially situational disturbances, mild tranquilization, i.e., Valium 5 or 10 mg PO or Ativan 1 or 2 mg PO might be helpful. If the patient is psychotic, treatment with neuroleptics could be of value, i.e., Navane, 10-15 mg, Haldol 5-10 mg may be given, concentrate or I.M. every 30 minutes. However, except for rare instances, *sedation should be avoided.* If the patient has overdosed, or if an overdose is suspected, then *medication should be avoided.*

D. It is important to realize that all suicide attempts are tinged with ambivalence and that once the patient comes to the emergency department the task of the physician is to support and encourage the patient that there are other ways to solve his problems. Instilling hope in the patient is the first step in shifting the patient's disposition towards life. If the suicidal patient cannot be seen immediately by a physician or psychiatrist, it is imperative not to leave him alone. If a sympathetic family member or friend is present he should be asked to sit with the patient; and in the event that the patient is alone, then a staff member should stay with the patient at all times.

E. A central issue in the treatment of a suicidal patient is educating the patient to other solutions for his problem. This is done by listening to the patient, providing guidance, interpretation, and education (e.g., a young woman makes a suicide attempt after she has seen her boyfriend with another woman. It might be helpful to point out other people that care for her, remind her she has had boyfriends before and most likely will have other boyfriends, and an interpretation of the component of her anger directed inward may be helpful).

F. The treating physician should attempt to increase the patient's feelings of being emotionally supported. This can be done by involving other significant persons in the patient's life. Bringing in spouses, lovers, or family friends will enhance the patient's feelings of being supported and cared for. When appropriate the feeling of support can further be enhanced by utilizing ancillary systems such as social services, job programs, welfare assistance programs and psychiatric outpatient and inpatient programs. The physician can also increase the patient's feelings of support by such statements as "I'm going to help you by giving medication to relax you, by making an appointment for you, by calling family, etc." The important statement is "I'm going to help."

G. When the patient does not respond to treatment, then the physician must decide whether to admit the patient. Generally, patients should be admitted as follows:

1. When a patient is psychotic.

2. When a patient is under the influence of drugs, especially hallucinogenic drugs.

3. When patients who are intoxicated present to an emergency room that is not equipped to hold them for 12 to 24 hours for observation.

4. When a patient must go home alone, and will be home by himself without supportive family or friends nearby.

5. When the suicidal ideation does not diminish and the patient's mood does not change despite the intervention of the physician, family, and/or friends.

If the examining physician is unsure of the suicidal risk, then it is better to err on the side of caution and admit the patient for at least 24 hours.

H. If the physician admits the patient, the following suicidal precautions should be taken:

1. If the patient is a high risk, there should be continuous observation, including when going to the bathroom, by a staff member, until the risk is reduced.

2. The patient should be placed in a hospital gown without ties; and sharp instruments, belts, and shoelaces should be removed. Stockings should be removed from the patient's room.

3. Agitated patients should be sedated and placed in restraints if necessary.

4. Patients on suicide precautions should be evaluated by a physician at least every six hours.

I. When a patient is discharged from the emergency department all efforts should be made to have friends or relatives accompany the patient home and spend the next 24 hours with him. Almost without exception, patients who presented with suicidal ideation or gestures should never be sent home alone. The patient should also be given the name and number of the treating physician and reassured that he can get in touch with the physician at any time. Ideally, the patient should have an outpatient appointment the following day.

References

1. Bellak, L. and Small, L. *Emergency Psychotherapy and Brief Psychotherapy,* 2nd edition. Grune and Stratton, New York, 1978.
2. Farberow, N.L. and Schneidman, E.S. *The Cry for Help.* McGraw-Hill, New York, 1965.
3. McKinnon, Roger A. and Michels, Robert. *The Psychiatric Interview in Clinical Practice.* W.B. Saunders, Philadelphia, 1971.
4. Schneidman, E.S. Psychotherapy with Suicidal Patients, Chapter 16

in *Specialized Techniques in Individual Psychotherapy,* edited by T.B. Karasu and L. Bellak. Brunner/Mazel, New York, 1980.

5. Sletten, I.W. and Barton, J.L. Suicidal Patients in the Emergency Room: A Guide for Evaluation and Disposition. *Hospital and Community Psychiatry.* V. 30, June, 1979, pp. 407–411.
6. Weiss, J.M.A. Suicide, Chapter 33 in *American Handbook of Psychiatry III,* edited by Silvano Arieti and Eugene B. Brody. Basic Books, New York, 1974, pp. 743–765.
7. Wolberg, L.R. *The Technique of Psychotherapy, Parts 1 and 2,* 2nd edition. Grune and Stratton, New York, 1967.

Chapter 8
Alcohol Abuse

Introduction

Alcohol abuse is a common and significant problem that is seen in the emergency room as either alcohol intoxication or alcohol withdrawal. Since intoxication and withdrawal can present as a medical and/or a behavioral emergency, treatment usually requires collaboration between the psychiatrist and the internist.

Alcohol Intoxication

A. *Acute Intoxication*—results from depression of the reticular activating system leading to cortical disinhibition with an acute stimulatory effect. A blood plasma alcohol level of 150 mg% is considered gross intoxication and levels above 500 mg% are potentially lethal. The intoxicated patient usually presents with symptoms of:

1. exhilaration and excitement
2. loss of restraint
3. slurred speech
4. incoordination of movements and gait
5. irritability
6. combativeness

7. drowsiness
8. signs of stupor and coma which include:
    a) decreased body temperature
    b) decreased respiratory rate
    c) stertorous breathing
    d) weak pulse
    e) contraction and dilation of pupils
    f) decreased or absent reflexes
    g) pale or cyanotic skin
    h) incontinence or retention of urine

Treatment

The treatment of the alcoholic patient begins with the initial interview and the course of the emergency room treatment can be influenced by the initial encounter between the physician and patient. In order to establish the most favorable treatment environment it is helpful for the examining physician to utilize the following techniques during the interview:

1. The interviewer should be tolerant and not threatening and should accept the intoxicated patient as he is, accepting insults and rudeness as part of the illness.

2. Coffee, food and support will often serve to calm the patient and make him more cooperative.

3. A physical examination is mandatory to rule out other medical conditions that may accompany alcoholic intoxication such as:
    a) Bleeding
    b) Cardiac arrhythmia
    c) Pneumonitis
    d) Head injury

4. The availability or presence of security personnel during the interview will often deter the belligerent patient from violent outbursts and will help to reassure the interviewer.

5. The patient is usually quieter if he is placed in a quiet room with minimal stimulation. He should be prevented from harming

himself and others. Soft physical restraints can be used when necessary.

6. Be cautious with alcoholics who are stuporous. Before letting them "sleep it off" make sure that they do not have a head injury or have overdosed with other drugs.

7. For sedating agitated patients, Librium 50-100 mg, p.o. or I.M., or Valium 10-20 mg p.o. or I.M. q 1-2 hrs is usually effective. Since absorption of intramuscular Valium and Librium can be erratic, it is preferable to try oral medication first. With extreme agitation, a high potency neuroleptic (Navane, Stelazine, Haldol) may be used (Ch. 6, p. 60).

8. Before definitive treatment can begin a differential diagnosis of diseases that may resemble alcohol intoxication must be considered. These include:
   a) intoxication with barbiturates or other sedative hypnotics
   b) multiple sclerosis
   c) Huntington's chorea
   d) hypoglycemia
   e) subdural hematoma
   f) cerebellar ataxia
   g) diabetic ketoacidosis

Disposition

1. The most preferable disposition is to send the patient home with supportive family or friends and refer the patient to an alcohol program the next day. Consider referral to Alcoholics Anonymous. Patients in this program have the lowest relapse rate.

2. If the above is not possible or if the patient needs to be observed longer, he should spend the night in the emergency department or be hospitalized. (No patient should be discharged who is ataxic.)

3. If the patient has an acute medical problem or has physically harmed other people or property, admission should be considered.

4. For management of patients with violent behavior, see Chapter 6.

5. Patients in an alcoholic coma are a medical emergency and require immediate intervention.

B. *Pathologic Intoxication*—is characterized by transitory, profound intoxication following the ingestion of small amounts of alcohol. Intoxication may be accompanied by an increase in aggressivity, depression, delusions, and disorientation. The patient is generally amnesic for the episode which lasts from a few minutes to several days. The emergency department treatment involves use of restraints and sedatives as needed. If the patient can be observed for several hours in the emergency room, hospitalization can usually be avoided. When medication is required for violent behavior, Navane 10-15 mg, Stelazine 10-15 mg, or Haldol 5-10 mg, concentrate or I.M. q 30 minutes may be helpful in tranquilizing the patient.

C. *Alcoholic Paranoia*—is found in patients with a long history of alcohol abuse. It occurs with intoxication and is manifested by:

1. Delusions of jealousy
2. Suspiciousness, anger, distrust
3. Ideas of reference
4. Occasional assaultiveness

These patients should be admitted to the hospital to be detoxified from alcohol and treated with neuroleptic medication.

D. *Chronic Intoxication*—may lead to the following sequelae:

1. Wernicke-Korsakoff's Syndrome which is characterized by ophthalmoplegia (diagnostic sign: ophthalmoplegia responds to thiamine within hours), nystagmus, impaired recent memory often resulting in confabulation, changes in mentation, most commonly a quiet delirium, peripheral neuritis and ataxia.
   a) *Treatment*—this condition requires immediate intervention since it is sometimes reversible. Treatment begins in the emergency department with Thiamine, 100 mg I.M. and should be continued giving 100 mg of Thiamine, I.M., T.I.D. for three days and then 100 mg, p.o. T.I.D. for 10 days. Patients should also be started on vitamin B complex

vitamins. The patient should be hospitalized and withdrawn from alcohol.

2. Alcoholic polyneuropathy is characterized by pain and muscle wasting. It occurs in alcoholics secondary to nutritional factors and is probably not related to the toxic effects of alcohol. Most patients are asymptomatic with loss of ankle and sometimes knee jerks. When symptoms occur, they consist of burning feet, pain, paresthesias, and mild distal weakness. The feet may be so sensitive that bed covers touching the feet are painful. In severe cases, the weakness may progress to wrist drop and foot drop.

   a) *Treatment* – the treatment consists of improving the diet and adding vitamin supplements. Recovery is slow but usually occurs with proper diet. Since polyneuropathy is nutritionally induced, the large majority of patients with Wernicke's syndrome have polyneuropathy as well.

3. Alcoholic amblyopia is a thiamine deficiency characterized by blurred vision, central scotomata, and papillitis. The treatment is Thiamine, 100 mg I.M. three times a day for 5 days then T.I.D. orally for 3 days.

4. "Schizophrenic-like" deterioration with cerebral and cerebellar atrophy. Intervention usually involves helping to control behavioral problems utilizing supportive therapy and neuroleptics.

5. Cerebellar degeneration is manifested by a history of an insidious onset of symptoms (weeks to months, though onset may be acute). Clinical symptoms include a wide-based gait, truncal instability and limb ataxia.

   a) *Treatment* – the treatment includes abstinence from alcohol, which is crucial, and dietary and vitamin support.

6. Seizures – Seizures can be precipitated by alcohol lowering the seizure threshold. Alcohol-induced seizures are usually focal and reflect an intrinsic CNS lesion. It is important to distinguish between seizures occurring when patient is intoxicated and withdrawal seizures. Patients who have seizures while drinking require basic neurological workup for a seizure disorder and treatment with anticonvulsants.

Alcohol Withdrawal States

A. A variety of symptoms and signs emerge when heavy and consistent drinkers suddenly stop or reduce their alcohol intake. In chronic alcoholics a minimum of a 2-week history of heavy drinking is necessary to develop a major abstinence syndrome. Well-known precipitants of withdrawal symptoms include severe physical stress such as pneumonitis or a major medical or surgical intervention which requires hospitalization and leads to a forced withdrawal.

The alcohol abstinence syndrome can be conceptualized as a release phenomenon from the depressant effects of alcohol. The excitatory activity of the CNS results in the following symptoms:

1. Hyperventilation
2. Tremulousness
3. Hyperreflexia
4. Withdrawal seizures
5. Psychomotor hyperactivity
6. Insomnia
7. Autonomic stimulation
8. Delirium

B. Classification of alcohol withdrawal states

1. *Minor Withdrawal*
   This phase consists of tremulousness and shakiness upon awakening after a night of abstinence from alcohol. Anxiety, muscle weakness, headache, anorexia, nausea and insomnia may occur. The morning-after sickness in binge or persistent alcohol abusers is actually an early, partial withdrawal syndrome.

2. *Impending Delirium Tremens* (DT's)
   The symptom complex of impending DT's includes shakiness, sweating and low grade fever. Agitation may occur and a mild degree of mental confusion may exist. Impending delirium tremens is the most common of the withdrawal syndromes. It can begin as early as 12 hours, or as late as 72 hours after the last drink. This condition will constitute the entire withdrawal experience for most patients.

a) *Treatment* – the treatment of the minor withdrawal syndrome or impending delirium tremens can be started in the emergency department and include:

- Tranquilization—50 to 100 mg of Librium orally or intravenously up to q 1 hour in the emergency department setting
- Thiamine, 100 mg intramuscularly
- Observation of patient for several hours in order to protect the patient and evaluate him for medical complications
- Mobilization of supportive resources such as family and friends
- Coffee and food will often help patient to relax.
- Medical evaluation
- Discharge patient with a 2-4 day prescription of Librium 100-200 mg in divided doses
- If possible, discharge the patient in the company of friends or relatives

b) Criteria for hospitalization of a patient withdrawing from alcohol include (from Shader, 1975):

- Delirium tremens
- Hallucinosis
- Seizure in patient with no known seizure disorder
- Presence of Wernicke's and/or Korsakoff's syndrome
- Fever over 101°F
- Head trauma with a period of unconsciousness
- Clouding of sensorium
- Presence of major medical illness, e.g., respiratory failure or infection, hepatic decompensation, pancreatitis, gastrointestinal bleeding, severe malnutrition
- Known history of delirium, psychosis, or seizures in previous untreated withdrawals

3. *Delirium Tremens*
   a) This is a late manifestation of alcohol withdrawal which peaks three to four days after cessation of drinking, but may be seen as late as ten days after last drink. Mortality has been

reported between 1% and 10%, with hyperthermia or peripheral vascular collapse as the usual causes of death. Symptoms include:

- Fluctuating delirium—worse during periods of reduced sensory input
- Visual and tactile hallucinations
- Marked confusion
- Disorientation
- Gross tremors which become worse when the patient is asked to perform an act
- Autonomic stimulation—high fever, tachycardia, hyperhidrosis, dilated pupils and elevated blood pressure

b) *Treatment*

- Medication will reduce CNS irritability. The drug of choice is Librium 100 mg p.o. q 4 hours which may be increased 1 gm/day if necessary. The dosage can be lowered gradually within one week. If the patient is extremely agitated and combative, use Navane 10–15 mg or Haldol 5–10 mg p.o. or I.M. q 1 hour until the patient is sedated.
- The presence of an electrolyte and/or water imbalance must be determined. Hypokalemia and hypomagnesemia are the most frequent electrolyte abnormalities.
- The physician should be alert for hypoglycemia, hepatic disease, head injuries and infections (especially pneumonia) which are common in alcoholics.
- Vitamin supplements include Thiamine, 100 mg I.M., T.I.D. for three days then 100 mg p.o. every day and multivitamins, one cap p.o. daily.
- Seizures—see Section 4.

4. *Alcoholic Seizures* ("Rum Fits")

Alcoholic seizures are generalized seizures which occur secondary to abstinence from alcohol or a reduction in usual intake. The onset is usually 12–48 hours after last intake. This *does not* represent a convulsive disorder. Characteristics include:

a) Seizures are grand-mal, non-focal and occur in groups of 2–3 and then stop.

b) EEG is normal.

c) Seizures do not require specific therapy unless repeated and life-threatening (status epilepticus).

Treatment:

a) There is no evidence that prophylactic treatment with Dilantin will prevent withdrawal seizures.

b) Candidates for emergency room treatment with Dilantin are patients with known underlying seizure disorder, who stopped taking Dilantin five or more days prior to admission. Treatment involves replacing the total body Dilantin stores with a loading dose of 1 gram in 250-500 cc's of 5% D_5W over 1-4 hours, then beginning maintenance therapy the following day (300-400 mg/day p.o.).

5. *Alcoholic Hallucinosis*

Alcoholic hallucinosis usually begins within a day after drinking has stopped and is characterized by an acute onset of auditory hallucinations. It may follow the impending delirium tremens, or it may appear without prodromal symptoms. It is distinguished from delirium tremens by the sensorium which is usually clear; orientation remains intact. Frequently the hallucinated voices make derogatory, accusatory or persecutory remarks about the listener and the patient responds to the voices as if they were real, e.g., a patient barricades his door because he hears the F.B.I. outside his door, planning to break into his room.

Treatment:

a) Hospitalization is usually necessary to protect the patient.

b) An adequate diet and vitamins are essential for proper nutritional care.

c) Reality orientation is important. Procedures should be explained to the patient and the room should be well lighted.

d) Neuroleptic medication can provide a useful adjunct to treatment; however, patient response is quite variable, and frequently medication has no effect on the hallucinations.

References

1. Cohen, S. Alcohol Withdrawal Syndromes, *Drug Abuse and*

Alcoholism Newsletter, Vistal Hill Foundation, San Diego, California, volume V, June 1976.

2. Greenblatt, D.J. and Shader, R.I. Treatment of the Alcohol Withdrawal Syndrome, in *Manual of Psychiatric Therapeutics,* edited by Richard I. Shader. Little, Brown and Co., Boston, 1975, pp. 211–235.

3. Hackett, T.P. Alcoholism: Acute and Chronic States in *Handbook of General Hospital Psychiatry,* edited by Hackett and Cassem. C.V. Mosby Co., St. Louis, 1978, pp. 15–28.

4. Madden, J.S. *A Guide to Alcohol and Drug Dependence.* John Wright and Sons, Bristol, England, 1979.

5. Slaby, A.E., Leib, J. and Tancredi, L.R. *Handbook of Psychiatric Emergencies,* 2nd edition. Medical Examination Publishing Company, Flushing, N.Y., 1980.

6. Victor, M. Alcoholism, Chapter 22 in *Textbook of Clinical Neurology,* edited by A.B. Baker. Harper and Row, Hagarstown, Maryland, 1978.

7. Wells, C.E. and Duncan, G.W. *Neurology for Psychiatrists.* F.A. Davis Co., Philadelphia, 1980.

8. Weiner, H.L. and Levitt, L.P. Neurology of Alcohol, in *Neurology for the House Officer,* 2nd edition. Williams and Wilkins Co., Baltimore, 1978, pp. 118–123.

Chapter 9
Drug Abuse

Introduction

This chapter is not intended to serve as a comprehensive guide to the medical treatment of drug overdoses. Comprehensive treatment requires a knowledge of general life support, and the specific treatment of various overdoses which includes knowledge of how to remove the poison, how to inactivate the poison, and finally what specific antidotes are available. For in depth reading on this topic, the authors recommend *Clinical Toxicology of Commercial Products* by Gosselin, et al. The presentation in this chapter will attempt to provide the physician with a basis for using the physical and psychological evaluation to make a reasonable assessment as to the type of drug intoxication or withdrawal that the patient is experiencing. The treatment approach will emphasize the management of the behavioral manifestations of toxicity with only a general outline of medical treatment.

In evaluating drug toxicity it must be remembered that etiologic diagnosis is often impossible to establish without laboratory analysis of a drug sample or of body fluids such as blood (10cc), urine (50-100cc) or stomach contents. Whenever possible, all three samples should be obtained. Even when the patient can "identify" the drug he has taken, most black market samples are characterized by four unknowns: dose, purity, actual identity and presence of contaminants. Concurrent illness or injury may complicate the clinical picture by augmenting the drug effect or failing to produce the usual symptoms. Despite the availability of laboratory analysis, the ability to make a clinical diagnosis based on signs and symptoms is important, since laboratory results frequently take hours to obtain. Furthermore, survival often depends on assessment and treatment in the first 30–60 minutes.

A general guideline for separating intoxications from withdrawals is the following:

1. Central Nervous System depression usually is indicative of intoxication, e.g., opiates, barbiturates, anti-anxiety agents. The major exception is stimulant drugs such as amphetamines, in which withdrawal can be characterized by lethargy and psychic depression.

2. The presence of restless or agitated behavior most commonly suggests the use of amphetamines, hallucinogens or withdrawal from barbiturates or opiates. Occasionally, marijuana can produce a similar reaction.

3. Helpful clinical clues for rapid assessment include:
    a) fever and psychosis suggest amphetamines or anticholinergic drugs
    b) dilated, unreactive pupils suggest anticholinergic drugs
    c) pinpoint pupils suggest opiates, except Demerol which may give dilated pupils.
    d) nystagmus and ataxia suggest barbiturates, anti-anxiety agents or Dilantin toxicity.

Drugs Producing Lethargy, Psychic Depression, or Coma

A. *Opiate Intoxication*

1. *Signs*
    a) pinpoint pupils unresponsive to light, except for Demerol which may produce dilated pupils.
    b) depressed respiration and level of consciousness
    c) bradycardia
    d) hypothermia
    e) pulmonary edema

TABLE I   Lethargy to Coma, Psychic Depression, Respiratory Depression

Drug	Blood Pressure	Temp.	Resp.	Pupils	G.I. Symptoms	Disorientation	Coma	Seizure	Tremors	Reflexes	Cardiac Arrhythmia	Resp. depression
Opiate intoxication	→	→	→	Pinpoint* Fixed	+		+					Pulmo-+ nary edema
Barbiturate intoxication	→	↑↓	→	Small-to-normal, reactive, nystagmus		+	+			→ Super-ficial		+
Non-barbiturate intoxication			Sudden Apnea	Doriden: miosis, followed by mydria-sis	+		+	+				+
Anti-anxiety agent intoxication							+	+				+

*Demerol may produce dilated pupils.

Treatment of Opiate Intoxication

The treatment of opiate intoxication is primarily medical. Naloxone (Narcan) is the antagonist of choice in the treatment of a narcotic overdose. It is used only to reverse severe respiratory depression and coma. The usual dose is 0.4 mg IV or I.M. every 3 minutes for a maximum of 3 doses. A treatment response can be noted by the patient becoming more arousable and the respiratory rate increasing to 10–12 per minute. In the event that no response occurs then another drug of abuse or another etiology for the depressed respiration and coma should be considered.

B. *Barbiturate Intoxication*

1. *Signs*
    a) Normal to small pupils, reactive to light (non-pinpoint)
    b) Nystagmus on lateral gaze
    c) Ataxia
    d) Slurred speech
    e) Confusion
    f) Decreased respiration and levels of consciousness
    g) Hypotension

2. *Treatment of Barbiturate Intoxication*
    The deaths that result from barbiturate and sedative ingestion are a result of cardiovascular and pulmonary depression. Therefore successful medical treatment involves supporting these systems. An airway should be established and suctioned when necessary. Blood pressure must be supported and vital signs frequently checked. Decisions concerning forced diuresis and dialysis are best left to senior medical residents and attending physicians.

C. *Intoxication with Non-Barbiturate Sedatives:* glutethimide (Doriden), meprobamate.(Equanil, Miltown)

1. *Signs*
    a) Similar to Barbiturates—See section B-1.
    b) *Doriden*
        Doriden poses a special problem when patients overdose and present in coma. Doriden is absorbed by the adipose tissues and is gradually released; therefore patients frequently wake up from a coma but will then lapse back into coma as more

of the drug is released from tissue stores. Other clinical findings in Doriden overdoses are contraction of pupils followed by dilation, sudden apnea, and acute laryngeal spasms.

2. *Treatment* —similar to treatment for barbiturate overdose. See Section B-2.

D. *Amphetamine Withdrawal*

1. Only considered an emergency when the patient is depressed and suicidal because of the withdrawal.

2. *Treatment*
   a) see Chapter 7, if suicidal.
   b) no gradual detoxification necessary.

E. *Anti-anxiety Agents (Benzodiazepine) Intoxication*

1. *Signs*
   a) confusion
   b) ataxia
   c) hypotension/shock
   d) slurred speech

2. *Treatment* —General medical support

Drugs Producing Restlessness or Agitation

A. *Opiate Withdrawal*

1. *Signs*
   a) Rhinorrhea—lacrimination
   b) G.I. disturbances
   c) sweating—piloerection
   d) restlessness and excitability
   e) muscle cramps

2. *Treatment*
   Opiate withdrawal is not a life-threatening situation. In order to keep the emergency room from being abused by opiate addicts,

TABLE II Restless Or Agitated

Drug	Blood Pressure	Temp.	Resp.	Pupils	G.I.	Disorientation	Coma	Seizure	Tremors	Reflexes	Cardiac Arrhythmia	Resp. depression
Opiate withdrawal	↑	↑	↑	Dilated reactive	++					↑		
Cocaine intoxication		↑	↑	Dilated	+		+	+	+	↑	+	+
Barbiturate withdrawal	↓	↑			+	+	+	+	+	↑		
LSD	↑			Dilated reactive		+	+	+	+	↑		
Amphetamine intoxication	↑	↑	Shallow	Dilated reactive	+	+		+	+	↑	+	+
PCP	↑			Constricted to normal, absent light reflex	+					Low doses ↑ High doses ↓		
Anticholinergic intoxication		↑		Dilated fixed	+	+		+		↑	+	+
Marijuana	↓			Injected conjunctiva	+						+	+

these patients should be referred to a methadone clinic. To give other drugs, such as minor tranquilizers, sedatives, and hypnotics is to encourage the patient to seek partial remedies and should be avoided. If the patient is in the hospital and requires methadone therapy, the clinic which the patient attends should be contacted to ascertain maintenance dose.

In general 10 mg of methadone given every 4-6 hours should be sufficient to prevent severe withdrawal.

B. *Barbiturate Withdrawal*

1. *Signs*
    a) tremors
    b) insomnia
    c) confusion and disorientation
    d) hallucinations
    e) hyperreflexia
    f) seizures

2. *Treatment* —(from Shader et al., 1975)
    a) Test dose: The patient is given 200 mg of pentobarbital orally and changes in the neurologic exam are assessed after one hour. The 24-hour pentobarbital requirement is estimated as follows:

Patient's condition one hour after test dose	Estimated 24-hour pentobarbital requirement (mg)
Asleep, but arousable	None
Drowsy, slurred speech; coarse nystagmus, ataxia, marked intoxication	400 to 600
Comfortable; fine lateral nystagmus is only sign of intoxication	800
No signs of drug effects; perhaps persisting signs of abstinence; no intoxication	1200 or more

If there are no signs of a drug effect, then the test is repeated three to four hours later using a dose of 300 mg of pentobarbital. No response to the 300 mg dose suggests a habit above 1600 mg per day.

b) Either pentobarbital or phenobarbital can be used for withdrawal, but phenobarbital has the advantage of few variations of blood barbiturate level. If pentobarbital is used, divide the estimated daily requirement into four equal doses and administer them every six hours. If phenobarbital is used, calculate dose at the rate of 30 mg of phenobarbital per each 100 mg of pentobarbital. Divide the total dose into three equal doses, and administer every eight hours.

c) Both pentobarbital and phenobarbital can be reduced at the rate of 10% per day.

d) *If concomitant addiction to opiate exists, barbiturate detoxification should proceed first, to be followed by opiate withdrawal at a later time.*

e) If seizures do occur, immediate treatment is with Valium 10 mg I.V. followed by Dilantin 1 gram in 250–500 cc's of 5% D_5W over 1–4 hours, then starting Dilantin 100 mg p.o. T.I.D. until the withdrawal process is completed.

f) With other non-barbiturate sedatives withdrawal is accomplished by gradual decrease in the abused drug.

g) Withdrawal from barbiturate is extremely dangerous and can result in seizures, cardiovascular collapse, and death. Therefore, barbiturate detoxification should be done in a hospital inpatient setting.

C. *Hallucinogens* (LSD, mescaline, psilocybin)

1. *Signs of intoxication:*
   a) Extreme, labile affect
   b) Dilated, although reactive, pupils
   c) Cyclical reactions and alternating periods of lucidness and intensive drug effect
   d) Perceptual distortion
   e) Most hallucinogens exert their major influence over 6–12 hours, but may last up to 24 hours or even several days.

2. *Common reactions to hallucinogens* – the most common presentation of hallucinogen intoxication is the:

   a) "Bad trip" – which is an adverse drug reaction following the use of hallucinogenic drugs for purpose of pleasure. Since self-harm is not the intent of drug use, it usually does not involve overdosage. Manifestations may vary from an acute panic reaction to a temporary psychotic state and include feelings of helplessness, fears of losing control, fears of going crazy, suspiciousness that can reach proportions of frank paranoia, intense anxiety, depression, and hallucinations, predominantly visual. LSD also causes sympathetic stimulation with pupillary dilation, diaphoresis and an increased pulse rate.

   b) *Treatment*

   - Reassurance is the most important therapeutic intervention. The patient should be told that the frightening feelings and perceptions are due to the drug he has taken and that he is not losing his mind. It is helpful to reassure the patient that the drug effects are temporary and that there will be no permanent damage from the drug. If the patient is disoriented, staff should continually orient the patient. Patients on bad trips should never be left alone. At times, their behavior can be life-threatening. Therefore, patients on bad trips should always be observed. Friends and family can often help staff not only to provide emotional support but can help staff to continuously monitor the patient.

      If medication is necessary then the drugs of choice are Valium 10 to 30 mg., p.o. or I.M. every 1 to 2 hours or Librium 25 to 100 mg. p.o. or I.M. until the patient has calmed down. Hospitalization is usually not necessary, but may be necessary if the reaction exceeds 24 hours despite vigorous intervention.

      All efforts should be made to avoid sending the patient home alone. Preferably he should be discharged in the custody of family or friends with an outpatient appointment the following day.

C. *Other common reactions are:*

1. "Flashback"—A flashback generally occurs in a patient that is a patient that is a chronic LSD user. It is a spontaneous recurrence of the original LSD trip and usually occurs suddenly and lasts several minutes though the reaction may last for several hours. The reaction is self-limiting and the treatment is the same as the treatment for bad trips.

D. *Amphetamine Intoxication*

1. *Signs*
   a) may mimic paranoid psychosis with the patient appearing to be schizophrenic
   b) increased blood pressure and respiration
   c) dilated, although reactive, pupils
   d) tachycardia
   e) fever
   f) respiratory failure
   g) seizures

2. *Treatment*
   a) The patient should be "talked down" by being given reassurance that the effects of the amphetamines will subside. Staff should not leave the patient alone and it is frequently helpful to have family and friends available to stay with the patient and also help provide reassurance and emotional support. Sensory stimulation should be minimized. If the patient is paranoid, the interviewer should avoid a confined setting which will make the patient feel overwhelmed. The interviewer should not move unnecessarily close to paranoid patients and he should stay at least an arm's length away.
   b) If symptoms are mild and patient is responsive to verbal instructions, benzodiazepines should be used in place of neuroleptics.
      - Valium 10–30 mg   p.o. preferably
        q 1-2 hrs   or
      - Librium 25–100 mg   I.M.
        q 1-2 hrs

c) In severely paranoid or agitated patients, neuroleptic medication is the treatment of choice. This may be given concentrate or I.M. as follows:

- Navane 10-15 mg every 30 minutes
- Stelazine 10-15 mg every 30 minutes
- Haldol 5-10 mg every 30 minutes

d) For severe adrenergic reactions (diaphoresis, tachycardia, hyperpyrexia, hypertension) the treatment of choice is Propranolol 20 to 40 mg p.o., or 1 to 2 mg intravenously except in asthmatics, diabetics and cardiovascular disease.

e) Hyperpyrexia is the most life-threatening complication and should be treated rigorously. *Any temperature greater than 102° is a medical emergency.* (Seizures are in the form of status epilepticus and should be treated with intravenous Valium 5 to 20 mg per minute and repeated at 15 minute intervals as necessary.)

f) If the paranoid behavior persists for longer than 12 hours, then hospitalization should be considered. The patient should be discharged to a responsible person who can observe the patient. An immediate outpatient appointment should also be made.

E. *Phencyclidine* (PCP)

Patients that present with PCP intoxication can be extremely combative and can pose a diagnostic and management problem. The signs of PCP intoxication include:

1. a florid psychosis that may be indistinguishable from schizophrenia
2. insensitivity to pain
3. disorientation
4. tachycardia
5. excessive salivation and diaphoresis
6. nystagmus and ataxia
7. hyperreflexia

Treatment
The psychological care of the patient with a PCP overdose is similar

to the care given the acutely psychotic patient (Chapter 4). Generally, the patient should be given reassurance that he will recover, and that his current thoughts and feelings are a result of the drug. External stimuli should be reduced and minimized and the patient should be spoken to in a soft non-threatening manner. Medication may be given as follows:

Valium:
2.5 mg at 10 minute intervals up to 25 mg, intravenously
or 5 mg increments up to 40 mg intramuscularly
or 10–20 mg orally

Patients with a PCP overdose must be closely monitored medically since large ingestions can result in coma and death. Vital signs, pulmonary and cardiovascular functioning must be observed and supported when necessary.

F. *Anticholinergic Intoxication* can occur from ingestion of atropine-like drugs, which include common over-the-counter sedatives (Compoz, Sleep-Eze, Sominex, etc.), and tricyclic antidepressants (Elavil, Tofranil, etc.). The signs of anticholinergic intoxication include:

1. dilated, unreactive pupils
2. dry mucous membranes
3. hot, dry, and flushed skin
4. hyperpyrexia
5. tachycardia, palpitations, elevated blood pressure
6. restlessness, excitement, confusion, delirium
7. hallucinations
8. arrhythmias
9. urinary/bowel retention
10. in rare instances, coma

Treatment
If the diagnosis is in doubt, then it is helpful to inject Metacholine, 10 to 30 mg subcutaneously. The failure of metacholine to elicit perspiration, salivation and rhinorrhea serves as a presumptive evidence of anticholinergic intoxication. A QRS duration of 100 milliseconds or more on routine EKG can be used to define a major overdose of antidepressants (Elavil,Tofranil, Sinequan, etc.).

The psychological treatment is similar to the treatment for delirium (Chapter 3). This involves reassurance, minimal sensory stimulation, and nursing supervision. Valium 5–10 mg I.M. or orally can be given for excitement. In the presence of uncontrollable agitation, cardiac arrhythmias, hypertension, or hyperpyrexia, physostigmine 1 to 2 mg I.M. or intravenously is the treatment of choice. When given intravenously, it is given at a rate of 1 mg per minute. If the symptoms recur, then physostigmine 1–4 mg I.M. or I.V. is repeated as necessary to control the agitation, arrhythmias, hypertension and hyperpyrexia. Physostigmine is relatively contraindicated in patients with diabetes, coronary artery disease, peptic ulcer, and ulcerative colitis.

Medical management also includes monitoring pulmonary functions and observing the patient for urinary retention.

G. *Marijuana Intoxication*

1. *Signs*
   a) euphoria, silliness, feeling of well-being
   b) rapid speech, talkativeness, flightiness
   c) altered space and time concepts
   d) increased appetite, thirst
   e) tachycardia, injected conjunctivae
   f) paranoid, anxious feelings

2. *Treatment*
   Treatment involves positive support and reassurance that the reaction is temporary. For anxiety, minor tranquilizers are the drugs of choice. Librium 20 mg initially, then 10 mg every hour to a total of 60 mg is effective for treating the tension and anxiety.

H. *Cocaine Intoxication*

1. *Signs*
   a) restlessness, excitability
   b) euphoria, hallucinations
   c) dilated pupils
   d) increased appetite, thirst
   e) convulsions, coma

    f)   rapid pulse followed by slow, weak pulse

    g)   paranoia

2. *Treatment*

Same as that for amphetamine abuse, see section on Drugs Producing Restlessness or Agitation, D 2.

I. *Methaqualone (Quaalude) Intoxication*

1. *Signs*
   a) restlessness
   b) delirium
   c) muscle spasms leading to convulsions and death
   d) most fatal doses involve a combination with alcohol
   e) it differs from barbiturate intoxication in that respiratory and cardiovascular depression are absent

2. *Treatment*

The treatment for Quaalude intoxication is medical and requires observation and, when necessary, support of vital life functions.

J. *Alcohol Withdrawal*

(see Chapter 8)

References

1. Biggs, J.T., Spiker, D.G., Petit, J.M. and Ziegler, V.E. Tricyclic Antidepressant Oversose. *JAMA*, 238(2):135–138, 1977.
2. Bourne, P.G. *A Treatment for Acute Drug Abuse Emergencies.* U.S. Department of Health, Education and Welfare, Rockville, Maryland, 1976.
3. Gosselin, R.E., Hodge, H.C., Smith, R.P. and Gleason, M.N. *Clinical Toxicology of Commercial Products,* 4th edition. Williams and Wilkins, Baltimore, 1976.
4. Greenblatt, D.J. and Shader, R.I. Drug Abuse and the Emergency Room Physician. *American Journal of Psychiatry,* 131:559–563, 1974.
5. Kline, N.S., Alexander, S.F., and Chamberlain, A. *Psychotropic Drugs: Manual for Emergency Management of Overdosage.* Medical Economics Company, Oradell, N.J., 1974.

6. Madden, J.S. *A Guide to Alcohol and Drug Dependence.* John Wright and Sons, Bristol, England, 1979.
7. Perry, P.J. and Juhl, R.P. Amphetamine Psychosis. *American Journal of Hospital Pharmacy,* 34:883–885, August 1977.
8. Rappolt, R.T., Gay, G.R. and Farris, R.D. Emergency Management of Acute Phencyclidine Intoxication. *JACEP,* 8:68–76, February, 1979.
9. Shader, R.I., Caine, E.D. and Meyer, R.E. Treatment of Dependence on Barbiturates and Sedative Hypnotics in *Manual of Psychiatric Therapeutics,* edited by R.I. Shader. Little, Brown and Co., Boston, 1975.
10. Shevitz, S. Emergency Management of the Agitated Patient. *Primary Care,* 5(4):625–634, 1978.

Chapter 10
Other Common Psychiatric Emergencies

Introduction

Complications of Neuroleptic Treatment

Patients being treated with neuroleptic medication often present to the emergency department with bizarre involuntary movements. These involuntary movements are usually extrapyramidal syndromes and are believed to result from the blockade of dopamine receptors in the basal ganglia. By eliciting a history of neuroleptic treatment, the physician can rapidly treat the patient and usually bring about immediate relief. Extrapyramidal symptoms fall into several discrete categories.

A. *Acute Dystonic Reaction* (ADR)

1. *Symptoms* — These reactions usually occur in the first few days of treatment with neuroleptic medication and result in spasms of the nuchal, truncal, or oculomotor muscle groups. ADRs frequently present as a torticollis or patients complaining of "my eyes rolling back in my head" — an oculogyric crisis. A very rare ADR, but one that can be fatal, is acute laryngeal spasms.

   The differential diagnosis of ADR includes seizure disorder, tetany, tetanus and, as it is most often diagnosed, hysteria. Generally ADR can be diagnosed in the presence of a history of treatment with neuroleptic drugs.

2. *Treatment*—Intramuscular or intravenous antiparkinson medication usually brings about rapid relief from the symptoms (3 to 5 minutes). The most frequently used drugs are:
   a) Benadryl 25 to 50 mg I.M. or I.V.—Recommended when a sedative effect is desired. Do not give Benadryl if the patient is alone or has to drive back home.
   b) Cogentin 2 mg I.M. or I.V.

   If the patient shows no response or only a partial response, repeat the dose in 15 minutes. A third dose may be tried, but generally if there is no response after 3 doses one should suspect another disease process (see above).

   Before discharge the patient should be placed on an antiparkinson agent and referred back to his psychiatrist for further evaluation. Maintenance drugs and doses include:

	usual dose range	starting dose
Benztropin (Cogentin)	1–6 mg/day	2 mg BID
Trihexyphenidyl (Artane)	5–15 mg/day	5 mg BID
Diphenhydramine (Benadryl)	25–100 mg/day	25 mg BID
Biperiden (Akineton)	2–6 mg/day	2 mg BID

B. *Akathisia*

1. *Symptoms*—Akathisia is a syndrome characterized by motor restlessness and an inability to sit still. The patient complains that he cannot sit still and must constantly keep walking. Frequently akathisia is mistaken for psychotic anxiety. A rough guide for distinguishing akathisia from psychotic anxiety has been outlined by Appleton and Davis (from Appleton, 1980). Differential points include:

Akathisia	Anxiety Agitation Psychotic Relapse
Driven by motor restlessness and unable to concentrate on voicing symptoms	Can concentrate on expressing symptoms at length

Symptoms primarily motor and cannot be controlled by the patient's will	Symptoms controllable
Worsened by dosage increase of neuroleptic medication	Relieved by dosage increase of neuroleptic medication
At times only responsiveness to antiparkinson agents distinguishes from anxiety or increased psychotic agitation	Unresponsive to antiparkinson agents

2. *Treatment*
   a) Antiparkinson agents may have a beneficial effect. Doses are generally the same as for dystonic reactions (Section A2).
   b) Unfortunately, akathisia does not always respond to antiparkinson agents and a failure to respond to antiparkinson medication does not rule out the presence of akathisia. Valium may have a beneficial effect. At times the only alternative to treating the akathisia is to decrease the dose of the neuroleptic medication or to change to a different neuroleptic.

C. *Drug-induced parkinsonism*

1. Resembles Parkinson's disease and symptoms include rigidity, drooling, mask-like facies, intention tremor, stooped posture, festinating gait and bradykinesia.

2. *Treatment* —Management involves prescribing antiparkinson drugs as noted in Section A-2.

D. *Other rare, acute toxic side effects to neuroleptic medication*

1. *Agranulocytosis*
   a) Usually occurs in first 8–16 weeks of treatment.
   b) Suspect in patients on neuroleptics who present with malaise, fever or sore throat.
   c) Stop medication *immediately* and obtain a CBC.
   d) The patient should have an immediate medical evaluation.

2. *Hypotension*
   a) If severe hypotension develops, this must be treated as a medical emergency.
   b) If a vasoactive agent is required the drugs of choice are alpha-adrenergic pressor amines — Metaraminol (aramine) 200 mg in 500cc of 5% D_5W.
   c) Beta-adrenergic drugs: *Isuprel and epinephrine are contraindicated.*

3. *Hypothalamic Crisis*
   a) Characterized by hyperthermia, sweating, drooling, tachycardia, dyspnea, seizures, unstable blood pressure.
   b) Creatinine phosphokinase may be extremely elevated and usually occurs in association with muscle rigidity.
   c) This is a medical emergency and requires immediate medical intervention.

Lithium Toxicity

A. Toxic effects of lithium can be seen at blood levels above 1.5 meq./L.Symptoms include:

1. muscle fasciculation and twitching
2. nystagmus
3. ataxia
4. somnolence, lethargy, coma
5. confusion
6. hyperactive deep tendon reflexes
7. dysarthria
8. rarely, seizures

B. *Treatment* —the main focus of treatment is to enhance lithium excretion by:

1. Replacing fluid and electrolytes as needed.
2. Forced diuresis with urea, 20 grams I.V., 2 to 5 times a day or mannitol 50–100 grams I.V. as a total daily dose.
3. Aminophylline-0.5 grams by slow I.V. increases lithium clearance.

4. Alkalinization of urine with sodium lactate.
5. If a diuretic is used, use a proximal tubule blocker, i.e., Diamox, since distal tubule blockers, i.e., thiazide or spironolactone, increase toxicity.
6. In severe poisoning, dialysis may be necessary.

Rape

A. Rape is a violent act. It is usually an act of aggression and hostility in which victims are often brutalized. When victims of rape arrive at the emergency department, they become patients with several important needs. As defined by Braen (1976) in *The Rape Examination* these needs include:

1. *Psychological needs*
   a) Minimization of psychological stress.
   b) Appropriate referral for follow-up.

2. *Medical needs*
   a) Immediate treatment of any physical stress.
   b) Evaluation for pregnancy and venereal disease.
   c) Appropriate referral for follow-up evaluation.

3. *Legal needs*
   a) Collection of medico-legal evidence.
   b) Maintenance of a legal record.
   c) Protection of the chain of evidence for police.

B. Psychological management of the rape victim:

1. The responses of victims vary widely from reactions of confusion, guilt, agitation and terror to some evidence of fear and anxiety. Some patients display complete calm and are even occasionally smiling. Since patients resent the offer of psychiatric help, immediate psychiatric intervention should be reserved for complicated cases or in dealing with difficult families.

2. *Staff attitude*—Psychological care begins the moment the patient arrives. Many myths about rape exist which lead people to

interpret rape in sexual terms rather than in terms of violence. As a result staff frequently have biased and ambivalent attitudes toward the victim. Any attitude which blames the victim will abort any chance for a therapeutic relationship. The staff should be non-judgmental and leave moral and legal judgment to others.

3. *Privacy* – The patient should have immediate attention and privacy. Consent forms for examination and future release of medical records should be obtained. Police officers *should not* be allowed in the examination room during the history and physical examination. Family members and friends should be discouraged from remaining in the examination room during the examination. However, a rape patient should never be left alone and preferably a female should be with the patient.

4. *Support* – Many patients will have the tendency to blame themselves for their handling of the rape encounter. The patient will need support and reassurance that whatever they did was appropriate because it helped them come out of this encounter alive. At times, patients will need to continuously repeat the story and will need constant reassurance and positive reinforcement. The most important task of the staff is to listen to the patient. Allowing the patient to share her feelings of pain, anger, guilt and embarrassment about the rape is the best therapy. Patients who are unwilling to talk about the experience and their feelings, even after being encouraged to do so, should be respected.

   The psychological sequelae of rape are unpredictable. Common preoccupations of patients which proper counselling in the emergency room can alleviate include: reassurance that they will have normal sexual relationships in the future though, initially, sexual relationships may be affected and that some degree of time, limited psychological distress, anxiousness, insomnia, etc. may occur. Finally, all rape patients should be made aware of appropriate counselling and treatment opportunities should the need arise in the future.

5. *The male rape victim* – The approach to the male rape victim is similar to the female victim. Aside from physical and anatomical differences, the psychological, medical, and legal issues are

similar. Male victims require the same staff attitude, privacy, and support as the female victim (Sec. A and B).

The medical and legal needs for rape victims require extensive discussion beyond the scope of this book. The optimal care requires a commitment of emergency department staff to all three areas of patients' needs.

References

1. Appleton, W.S. and Davis, J.M. *Practical Clinical Psychopharmacology,* 2nd Edition. Williams and Wilkins, Baltimore, 1980.
2. Baldessarini, R.J. *Chemotherapy in Psychiatry.* Harvard University Press, Cambridge, Mass., 1977.
3. Braen, G.R. *The Rape Examination.* Abbott Laboratories, Chicago, Illinois, 1976.
4. Burgess, A.W. and Holmstrom, L.L. Rape Trauma Syndrome. *American Journal of Psychiatry,* 131:981–987, 1974.
5. Burgess, A.W. and Holmstrom, L.L. The Rape Victim in the Emergency Ward. *American Journal of Nursing,* 73:1741–1745, 1973.
6. Detre, T.O. and Jarecki, H.G. Psychotropic Agents, chapter 14 in *Modern Psychiatric Treatment,* J.B. Lippincott Co., Philadelphia, 1971, pp. 542–591.
7. Falk, N. Clinical Management of Rape. *Hospital Physician,* June, 1977, pp. 34–38.
8. Josephson, G.W. The Male Rape Victim: Evaluation and Treatment. *Journal of the American College of Emergency Physicians,* 8:13–15, 1979.
9. Nadelson, C.C. and Notman, M.T. Psychological Responses to Rape. *Psychiatry Opinion,* July/August, 1977, pp. 13–18.

Appendix
PSYCHIATRIC SIDE EFFECTS OF MEDICAL DRUGS

PSYCHIATRIC SIDE EFFECTS OF MEDICAL DRUGS

General Classification	Generic	Trade Name	Psychiatric Side Effects

Sulfonamides*	Mafenide acetate
	Phthelylsulfathiazole
	Salicylazosulfapyridine
	Sulfacetamide sodium
	Sulfachlorpyridazine
	Sulfadiazine
	Sulfamerazine
	Sulfameter
	Sulfamethazine
	Sulfamethizole
		Sulfamylon
		
		Sultrin Triple Sulfa
		
		Suladyne
		
		Sulla
		
		Azotrex
		Microsul
		Microsul-A
		Suladyne
		Thiosulfil
		Thiosulfil Forte
		Thiosulfil-A Forte
		Urobiotic-250
			General statement regarding
			sulfonamides:
			  depression
			  psychosis
			  restlessness
			  irritability
			
			*May cause retardation if given
			during 3rd trimester, to nursing
			mothers, or to children less than
			2 months old

	Sulfamethoxazole	Azo Gantanol Bactrim DS Bactrim Gantanol Gantanol DS Septra DS Septra	
	Sulfaphenasole Sulfisoxazole	Azo Gantrisin Gantrisin SK-Soxazole Sulfisoxazole Vagilia	

PSYCHIATRIC SIDE EFFECTS OF MEDICAL DRUGS (Cont.)

General Classification	Generic	Trade Name	Psychiatric Side Effects
Sulfones	Dapsone Sulfoxone sodium		General statement regarding sulfones: nervousness insomnia psychosis
Anthelmintics	Aspidium oleoresin Quinacrime HCl Tetrachloroethylene	Male Fern Oleoresin Atabrine HCl	Delirium Psychosis Inebriation
Antitubercular Agents	Cycloserine	Seromycin	Confusion Lethargy Psychosis
	Ethionamide Isoniazid	Trecator-SC INH Isonicotinic Acid Hydrazine Hyzyd Laniazid Niconyl Nydrazid Teebaconin	Depression Toxic psychosis Parasthesia Excitement Euphoria
	Rifampin	Rifadin Rimactane	Confusion
Antimalarials	Chloroquine HCl Chloroquine phosphate	Aralen HCl Aralen Phosphate	General statement regarding antimalarials: fatigue lassitude nervousness irritability psychosis
	Amodiaquin HCl	Camoquin HCl	Spasticity

PSYCHIATRIC SIDE EFFECTS OF MEDICAL DRUGS (Cont.)

General Classification	Generic	Trade Name	Psychiatric Side Effects
Amebicides and Trichomonacides	Metronidazole	Flagyl	Confusion Irritability Depression Insomnia
Antineoplastic Agents	Fluorouracil	Efudex 5-Fluorouracil 5-FU Fluoroplex	Euphoria Insomnia Irritability
	Procarbazine HCl	Matulane	Depression Psychosis Manic reactions Nervousness Insomnia Nightmares Disorientation Delirium
	Vinblastine sulfate	Velban VLB	Depression
Cardiac Glycosides	Acetyldigitoxin Deslanoside Digitalis glycoside Digitalis leaf Digitoxin Digoxin Gitalin Lanatoside C Ouabain	Acylanid Cedilanid-D Crystodigin Digitoxin Digoxin Lanoxin SK-Digoxin Gitaligin Cedilanid Ouabain	General statement regarding cardiac glycosides: disorientation confusion depression aphasia delirium hallucinations especially in the elderly or arteriosclerotic

PSYCHIATRIC SIDE EFFECTS OF MEDICAL DRUGS (Cont.)

General Classification	Generic	Trade Name	Psychiatric Side Effects
Peripheral Vasodilators	Nylidrin HCl	Nylidrin Arlidin	Nervousness
Antihypertensive Agents			
Rauwolfia Alkaloids	Alseroxylon Deserpidine	Enduronyl Harmonyl Oreticyl	General statement regarding Rauwolfia alkaloids: nightmares depression (to point of suicide attempt)
	Rauwolfia serpentina	Raudixin Rauzide Rauwolfia Serpentine	Rare: nervousness, paradoxical anxiety, decreased libido, Parkinson-like syndrome
	Rescinnamine Reserpine	Moderil Butiserpazide-25/50 Prestabs Demi-Regroton Diupres Diutensen-R Dralserp Exna-R Hydromox R Hydropres Hydrotensin-50 Hydrotensin-Plus Metatensin Naquival Ran-Sed Regroton Renese-R Reserpine Ruhexatal with reserpine SK-Reserpine	

PSYCHIATRIC SIDE EFFECTS OF MEDICAL DRUGS (Cont.)

General Classification	Generic	Trade Name	Psychiatric Side Effects
Rauwolfia Alkaloids (Cont.)	Reserpine (Cont.)	Salutensin Sandril Ser-Ap-Es Serpasil Serpasil-Apresoline Serpasil-Esidrix Singoserp-Esidrix	
	Syrosingopine		
Ganglionic Blocking Agents	Mecamylamine HCl Pentolinium tartrate Trimethaphan camsylate	Arfonad	General statement regarding ganglionic blocking agents: tremor confusion
Sympathetic Nervous System Depressants	Guanethidine sulfate Methyldopate HCl	Ismelin Sulfate Aldomet HCl	Depression Parkinsonism Diminished cognition Choreoathetotic movements Nightmares Depression Psychosis
	Methyldopa	Aldomet Aldoclor Aldoril	Parkinsonism Diminished cognition Choreoathetotic movements Nightmares Depression Psychosis
Agents that Act Directly on Vascular Smooth Muscle	Hydralazine HCl	Apresazide Apresoline HCl Apresoline-Esidrix	Depression Disorientation Anxiety

PSYCHIATRIC SIDE EFFECTS OF MEDICAL DRUGS (Cont.)

General Classification	Generic	Trade Name	Psychiatric Side Effects
Agents that Act Directly on Vascular Smooth Muscle (Cont.)	Hydralazine HCl (Cont.)	Dralserp Dralzine Hydralazine HCl Hydrotensin-Plus Ser-Ap-Es Serpasil-Apresoline Unipres	
Antiarrhythmic Agents	Lidocaine HCl	Anestacon LTA 11 Lidocaine HCl Lidosporin Xylocaine HCl	Transient excitement Depression Restlessness Euphoria Apprehension Hallucinations Insomnia Incoordination
	Propranolol HCl	Inderal	
Hypocholesterolemic and Antilipemic Agents	Nicotinic acid	Cerebro-Nicin Diacin Lipo-Nicin Menic Niac Niacin Nicalex Nicobid Nicocap Nico-400 Nicolar Nico-Metrazol	Nervousness Panic reactions

PSYCHIATRIC SIDE EFFECTS OF MEDICAL DRUGS (Cont.)

General Classification	Generic	Trade Name	Psychiatric Side Effects
Hypocholesterolemic and Antilipemic Agents (Cont.)	Nicotinic acid (Cont.)	Nico-Span Nicotinex Elixir Nicozol Progiatric Ragus Tega-Span Tinic Wampocap	
	Dextrothyroxine sodium	Choloxin	Insomnia Nervousness Changes in libido ($>$ or $<$) Bizarre subjective complaints

Barbiturates	Amobarbital	Amesec
		Amytal
		Dexamyl
		Ectasule
			General statement regarding barbiturates:
			  excitement
			  euphoria
			  restlessness
			  delirium

	Amobarbital sodium	Amytal Sodium Tuinal	
	Aprobarbital	A.P.B. Alurate Elixir Alurate Elixir Verdum	psychological dependence nervousness
	Butabarbital	Broncomar Butabarbital Sodium Elixir Butiserpazide-25/50 Cystospaz-SR Dolonil Quibron Plus Sedapap-10 Sidonna Tedral-25	

PSYCHIATRIC SIDE EFFECTS OF MEDICAL DRUGS (Cont.)

General Classification	Generic	Trade Name	Psychiatric Side Effects
Barbiturates (Cont.)	Butabarbital sodium	Buticaps	
		Butisol	
		Dularin-TH	
		Gaysal	
		Minotal	
		Phrenilin	
	Hexobarbital	Mebaral	
	Mephobarbital	Gemonil	
	Metharbital		
	Methhexital sodium		
	Pentobarbital	Eme-Nil Inserts	
		Emesert Inserts	
		Matropinal	
		Matropinal Forte	
		Nembutal Elixir	
		Pentobarbital Sodium	
	Phenobarbital	A.P.B.	
		Antrocol	
		Arco-Lase Plus	
		Belap	
		Bentyl with Phenobarbital	
		Bronkolixir	
		Bronkotabs	
		Bronkotabs-Hafs	
		Cantil with Phenobarbital	
		Cardilate-P	
		Donphen	
		Eskabarb	
		Gaysal	
		Gustase-Plus	
		Isordil	

PSYCHIATRIC SIDE EFFECTS OF MEDICAL DRUGS (Cont.)

General Classification	Generic	Trade Name	Psychiatric Side Effects
Barbiturates (Cont.)	Phenobarbital (Cont.)	Levsin/Phenobarbital	
		Levsinex/Phenobarbital	
		Lufyllin-EPG	
		Luminal	
		Matropinal	
		Mundrane GG	
		Oxoids	
		Pamine PB	
		Peritrate with Phenobarbital	
		Phazyme-PB	
		Phenobarbital	
		Pro-Banthine with Phenobarbital	
		Proval	
		Quadrinal	
		Robinul with Phenobarbital	
		SK-Phenobarbital	
		Solfoton	
		Trasentine with Phenobarbital	
		Valpin	
		Verequad	
	Phenobarbital sodium	Luminal Sodium	
	Secobarbital	Antora-B	
		Secobarbital	
		Seconal Elixir	
	Secobarbital sodium	Seconal Sodium	
	Talbutal	Lotusate	
	Thiamylal sodium	Surital Sodium	
	Thiopental sodium	Pentothal Sodium	

PSYCHIATRIC SIDE EFFECTS OF MEDICAL DRUGS (Cont.)

General Classification	Generic	Trade Name	Psychiatric Side Effects
Nonbarbiturate sedatives and hypnotics	Bromide salts	Sodium	Bromide psychosis
		Potassium	Depression
		Ammonium	
	Bromide salts, mixed	Neurosine	Depression
			Bromide psychosis
	Bromisovalum	Bromural	Bromide psychosis
	Chloral hydrate	Aquachloral	Paranoid reactions
		Chloral Hydrate	Chloral delirium
		Cohydrate	
		Felsules	
		Kessodrate	Somnambulism
		Lycoral	
		Noctec	
		Oradrate	
		Rectules	
		SK-Chloral Hydrate	
		Somnos	
	Ethinamate	Valmid	Paradoxical excitement in children
	Glutethimide	Doriden	Psychosis
		Glutethimide, NF	Confusion
			Delirium
			Hallucinations
	Methyprylon	Noludar	Paradoxical excitement
			Confusion

PSYCHIATRIC SIDE EFFECTS OF MEDICAL DRUGS (Cont.)

General Classification	Generic	Trade Name	Psychiatric Side Effects
Anticonvulsants			

Hydantoins	Diphenylhydantoin	Dihycon
		Dilantin
		DPH
		Ekko
		Phenytoin
		Toin Unicelles
			General statement regarding hydantoins:
			  hallucinations
			  delusions
			  extrapyramidal reactions

	Diphenylhydantoin sodium	Dilantin Sodium Kessodanten Phenytoin Sodium	
	Ethotoin Mephenytoin	Peganone Mesantoin	Confusion Psychosis Irritability Depression

Succinimides	Ethosuximide
	Phensuximide
		Zarontin
		Milontin
			General statement regarding succinimides:
			  nervousness
			  apathy
			  euphoria
			  depression
			  personality change
			  confusion
			  severe depression

	Methsuximide	Celontin	
Miscellaneous	Phenacemide	Phenurone	Psychosis with suicidal tendencies Depression Aggressiveness

PSYCHIATRIC SIDE EFFECTS OF MEDICAL DRUGS (Cont.)

General Classification	Generic	Trade Name	Psychiatric Side Effects
Miscellaneous (Cont.)	Primidone	Mysoline	Irritability Hyperexcitability (particularly in children)
Narcotic analgesics			
Morphine and Congeners	Codeine	Calcidrine Syrup Empracet with Codeine Promethazine HCl Expectorant with Codeine Pyribenzamine Expectorant with Codeine & Ephedrine SK-APAP with Codeine	General statement regarding morphine and congeners: mental clouding euphoria excitement restlessness delirium insomnia
	Codeine phosphate	APC with Codeine Actifed-C Ascodeen-30 Ascriptin with Codeine Bancap with Codeine Capital with Codeine Chlor-Trimeton Expectorant with Codeine Codalan Codimal PH Colrex Compound Dimetane Expectorant-DC Empirin Compound with Codeine Emprazil-C Fiorinal with Codeine Isoclor Expectorant Novahistine DH Novahistine Expectorant	

PSYCHIATRIC SIDE EFFECTS OF MEDICAL DRUGS (Cont.)

General Classification	Generic	Trade Name	Psychiatric Side Effects
Morphine and Congeners (Cont.)	Codeine phosphate (Cont.)	Nucofed Syrup	
		Pediacof	
		Phenaphen with Codeine	
		Phenergan Expectorant with Codeine	
		Proval #3	
		Robitussin A-C	
		Robitussin DAC	
		Ryna-C Syrup	
		Ryna-CX Syrup	
		Sinutab with Codeine	
		Soma Compound with Codeine	
		Triaminic Expectorant with Codeine	
		Tussi-Organidin	
		Tylenol with Codeine	
	Codeine Sulfate	Copavin	
	Fentanyl	Innovar	
		Sublimaze	
	Hydromorphone	Dilaudid	
	Levorphanol tartrate	Levo-Dromoran	
	Methadone HCl	Dolophine HCl	
		Vitarine	
		Westadone	
	Morphine sulfate		
	Opium preparations	B&O Supprettes No. 15A & 16A	
		BPP-Lemmon	
		Donnagel PG	
		Pantopon	
		Parepectolin	

PSYCHIATRIC SIDE EFFECTS OF MEDICAL DRUGS (Cont.)

General Classification	Generic	Trade Name	Psychiatric Side Effects
Morphine and Congeners (Cont.)	Oxycodone	Percocet-5 Percodan Tylox	
	Oxymorphone Pentazocaine	Numorphan HCl Talwin	Dysphoria Nightmares Hallucinations Psychological dependence
Meperidine and Congeners	Alphaprodine HCl Anileridine Meperidine HCl	Nisentil HCl Leritine Demerol	General statement regarding Meperidine and Congeners: dysphoria agitation euphoria transient hallucinations disorientation
Miscellaneous Analgesics	Methotrimeprazine	Levoprome	Delirium Extrapyramidal symptoms
Narcotic Antagonists	Levallorphan tartrate	Lorfan	Dysphoria Bizarre or unusual dreams Visual hallucinations Disorientation Derealization
	Nalorphine HCl	Nalline HCl	Dysphoria Psychotomimetic manifestations

PSYCHIATRIC SIDE EFFECTS OF MEDICAL DRUGS (Cont.)

General Classification	Generic	Trade Name	Psychiatric Side Effects
Cerebral and Respiratory Stimulants			
Amphetamines and Derivatives	Amphetamine sulfate	Delcobese Fetamin Obetrol	General statement regarding amphetamines and derivatives: paradoxical increased depression & agitation in depressed patients depression disorientation hallucinations
	Benzphetamine HCl Chlorphentermine HCl	Didrex Pre-Sate	Psychic dependence
	Dextroamphetamine sulfate	Dexamyl Dexedrine Dextro-Amphetamine Eskatrol	Paranoia Schizophreniform psychosis
	Dextroamphetamine tannate	Obotan Obotan Forte	
	Diethylpropion HCl	Tenuate Dospan Tenuate 25 Tepanil Tepanil Ten-Tab	
	Methamphetamine HCl	Desoxyn Fetamin	
	Phendimetrazine tartrate	Bacarate Banobese Bontril PDM Melfiat Phendiet Plegine	

PSYCHIATRIC SIDE EFFECTS OF MEDICAL DRUGS (Cont.)

General Classification	Generic	Trade Name	Psychiatric Side Effects
Amphetamines and Derivatives (Cont.)	Phendimetrazine tartrate (Cont.)	Statobex Statobex-G Trimstat Trimtabs	
	Phenmetrazine HCl	Phendimetrazine bitartrate Preludin Endurets Preludin	
	Phentermine HCl	Adipex 8 Adipex-P Fastin Phentercot T.D. Ionamin	
	Phentermine resin		
Miscellaneous Agents	Methylphenidate HCl	Ritalin HCl	Nervousness Insomnia Psychological dependence
Nonnarcotic Analgesics and Antipyretics			
Salicylates	Acetylsalicyclic acid Calcium carbaspirin	Fiogesic Ursinus Inlay-Tabs	General statement regarding salicylates:
	Choline salicylate	Arthropan Trilisate	emotional disturbances that mimic alcohol inebriation.
	Magnesium salicylate	Hyalex Lorisal Magan Mobidin Trilisate	hyperventilation agitation confusion

PSYCHIATRIC SIDE EFFECTS OF MEDICAL DRUGS (Cont.)

General Classification	Generic	Trade Name	Psychiatric Side Effects
Salicylates (Cont.)	Methylsalicylate Salicylamide	Arthralgen Bancap Bancap with Codeine Codalan Coriforte Excedrin Excedrin P.M. Os-Cal-Gesic Rhinex D-Lay Sinulin	
	Sodium salicylate	Corilin Gaysal Gaysal-S Pabalate	
Para-Aminophenol Derivatives	Acetaminophen	APAP Acetaminophen Anuphen Suppositories Arthralgen Bancap Bancap with Codeine Capital Capital with Codeine Codalan Colrex CoTylenol Darvocet Datril Demerol APAP Dialog	General statement regarding para-aminophenol: confusion excitement delirium psychological dependence

PSYCHIATRIC SIDE EFFECTS OF MEDICAL DRUGS (Cont.)

General Classification	Generic	Trade Name	Psychiatric Side Effects
Para-Aminophenol Derivatives (Cont.)	Acetaminophen (Cont.)	Dularin-TH	
		Duradyne DHC	
		Empracet with Codeine	
		Esgic	
		Excedrin	
		Excedrin P.M.	
		Febrigesic	
		Gaysal	
		Gaysal-S	
		Liquiprin	
		Midrin	
		Minotal	
		Nebs Analgesic	
		Ornex	
		Parafon Forte	
		Percocet-5	
		Percogesic	
		Phenaphen	
		Phenaphen with Codeine	
		Phrenilin	
		Proval #3	
		Repan	
		Rhinex D-Lay	
		SK = APAP	
		SK = APAP with Codeine	
		SK = 65 APAP	
		Sedapap-10	
		Sinarest	
		Singlet	
		Sinubid	
		Sinulin	

PSYCHIATRIC SIDE EFFECTS OF MEDICAL DRUGS (Cont.)

General Classification	Generic	Trade Name	Psychiatric Side Effects
Para-Aminophenol Derivatives (Cont.)	Acetaminophen (Cont.)	Sinutab	
		Sinutab II	
		Sinutab with Codeine	
		Sunril	
		Supac	
		Tempra	
		Trind	
		Trind-DM	
		Tussagesic	
		Tylenol	
		Tylenol Extra Strength	
		Tylenol with Codeine	
		Tylox	
		Valadol	
		Vanquish	
		Wygesic	
	Phenacetin (acetophenetidin)	A.P.C.	
		A.P.C. with Codeine	
		A.P.C. with Butalbital	
		Buff-A Comp	
		Buffadyne-Lemmon	
		Empirin	
		Empirin with Codeine	
		Emprazil	
		Emprazil-C	
		Fiorinal	
		Fiorinal with Codeine	
		Monacet (APC) with Codeine	
		Norgesic	
		SK-65 Compound	

PSYCHIATRIC SIDE EFFECTS OF MEDICAL DRUGS (Cont.)

General Classification	Generic	Trade Name	Psychiatric Side Effects
Para-Aminophenol Derivatives (Cont.)	Phenacetin (acetophenetidin) (Cont.)	Soma Soma with Codeine Synalgos Synalgos-DC	
Miscellaneous Agents	Fenoprofen calcium	Nalfon	Confusion Nervousness Insomnia
	Indomethacin	Indocin	Confusion Depression Psychosis
	Naproxen	Naprosyn	Depression
	Propoxyphene HCl	Darvon Darvon-ASA Dolene Harmar Progesic-65 Propoxychel Propoxyphene Compound 65 Propoxyphene HCl APAP Propoxyphene HCl with APC Proxagesic SK-65 Stero-Darvon with ASA Unigesic-A Wygesic	Decreased concentration Euphoria Dysphoria Psychological dependence
	Tolmetin sodium	Tolectin	Tension Nervousness

PSYCHIATRIC SIDE EFFECTS OF MEDICAL DRUGS (Cont.)

General Classification	Generic	Trade Name	Psychiatric Side Effects
Adrenergic (Sympathomimetic) Drugs			
	Dopamine HCl	Intropin	General statement regarding adrenergic drugs:
	Ephedrine	Amesec	excess stimulation
		Bronkolixir	insomnia
		Bronkotabs	restlessness
		Bronkotabs-Hafs	nervousness
		I-Sedrin Plain	tremor
		Pyribenzamine with Codeine and Ephedrine	
		Pyribenzamine with Ephedrine	
		Quibron Plus	
	Ephedrine HCl	Bronchobid Duracap	
		Calcidrine Syrup	
		Derma Medicone-HC	
		KIE	
		Lufyllin-EPG	
		Mudrane GG	
		Mudrane	
		Quadrinal	
		Quelidrine Syrup	
		Tedral	
		Tedral SA	
		Tedral-25	
		Verequad	
	Ephedrine lactate	Gluco-Fedrin	
	Ephedrine sulfate	Ectasule Minus	
		Ephed-Organidin	
		Isuprel Compound	
		Marax	
		Pazo Ointment	
		Slo-Fedrin	

PSYCHIATRIC SIDE EFFECTS OF MEDICAL DRUGS (Cont.)

General Classification	Generic	Trade Name	Psychiatric Side Effects
Adrenergic (Sympathomimetic) Drugs (Cont.)			
	Epinephrine	Adrenalin Chloride	
		Asmolin	
		Asthma-meter	
		Primatene Mist	
		Sus-phrine	
	Epinephrine bitartrate	Asmatane	
		Medihaler-Epi	
		Epitrate Opthalmic	
		Lyophrin Opthalmic	
		Mytrate Opthalmic	
	Ephinephrine borate	Epinal Opthalmic	
		Eppy Opthalmic	
	Ephinephrine HCl	Adrenaline HCl	
		Vaponefrin	
		Epifrin Opthalmic	
		Glaucon Opthalmic	
		Mistura E Opthalmic	
	Ethylnorepinephrine HCl	Bronkephrine	
	Hydroxyamphetamine hydrobromide	Paredrine	
	Isoproterenol HCl	Aerolone Compound	
		Duo-Medihaler	
		Iprenol	
		Isuprel	
		Norisodrine Aerotrol	
		Norisodrine with Calcium Iodide	
		Vapo-N-Iso	

PSYCHIATRIC SIDE EFFECTS OF MEDICAL DRUGS (Cont.)

General Classification	Generic	Trade Name	Psychiatric Side Effects
Adrenergic (Sympathomimetic) Drugs (Cont.)	Isoproterenol sulfate	Iso-Autohaler	
		Luf-Iso	
		Medihaler-Iso	
		Norisodrine Sulfate	
	Levarterenol bitartrate	Levophed Bitartrate	
		Norepinephrine Bitartrate	
	Mephentermine sulfate	Wyamine Sulfate	
	Metaraminol bitartrate	Aramine Bitartrate	
		Pressonex Bitartrate	
	Methoxamine HCl	Vasoxyl	
	Methoxyphenamine HCl	Orthoxine	
	Nylidrin HCl	Arlidin HCl	
	Phenylephrine HCl	Chlor-Trimeton	
		Chlor-Trimeton with Codeine	
		Citra	
		Citra Forte	
		Codimal DH	
		Codimal DM	
		Codimal PH	
		Coltrex Compound	
		Congespirin	
		Coricidin	
		Coricidin Demilets	
		Coryban-D	
		Dallergy	
		Demazin	
		Dimetane	
		Dimetane DC	
		Dimetapp	
		Dimetapp Extentabs	
		Entex	

PSYCHIATRIC SIDE EFFECTS OF MEDICAL DRUGS (Cont.)

General Classification	Generic	Trade Name	Psychiatric Side Effects
Adrenergic (Sympathomimetic) Drugs (Cont.)	Phenylephrine HCl (Cont.)	Extendryl	
		4-Way Nasal Spray	
		Guistrey Fortis	
		Histalet Forte	
		Histaspan-D	
		Histaspan-Plus	
		Histatapp	
		Histatapp TD	
		NTZ	
		Naldecon	
		Napril Plateau Caps	
		Narine Gyrocaps	
		Neo-Synephrine	
		Ocusol Opthalmic	
		Oraminic Spancap	
		Pediacof	
		Phenergan VC	
		Phenergan VC with Codeine	
		Puretapp	
		Puretapp PA	
		Quelidrine	
		Respinol-G	
		Rhinex	
		Ryna-Tussadine	
		S-T Forte	
		Singlet	
		Trind	
		Trind-DM	
		Tussanil DH	
		Tympagesic	

PSYCHIATRIC SIDE EFFECTS OF MEDICAL DRUGS (Cont.)

General Classification	Generic	Trade Name	Psychiatric Side Effects
Adrenergic (Sympathomimetic) Drugs (Cont.)	Phenylpropanolamine HCl	Allerest	
		Allerest Timed Release	
		Anorexin	
		Bayer Children's Cold Tablets	
		Codimal	
		Coricidin	
		Coricidin "D"	
		Coryban-D	
		Cotofed	
		Decongest TD	
		Dibron	
		Dimetane	
		Dimetane-DC	
		Dimetapp	
		Dimetapp Extentabs	
		Dorcol	
		Entex	
		Fiogesic	
		Histabid Duracap	
		Histalet Forte	
		Histatapp	
		Histatapp T.D.	
		Hycomine	
		Korigesic	
		Kronohist Kronocaps	
		MSC Triaminic	
		Naldecon	
		Napril Plateau	
		Nolamine	
		Novahistine	
		Novahistine DH	

PSYCHIATRIC SIDE EFFECTS OF MEDICAL DRUGS (Cont.)

General Classification	Generic	Trade Name	Psychiatric Side Effects
Adrenergic (Sympathomimetic) Drugs (Cont.)	Phenylpropanolamine HCl (Cont.)	Ornacol	
		Ornade	
		Ornex	
		Puretapp	
		Puretapp-PA	
		Respinol-G	
		Rhinex D-Lay	
		Rhinex DM	
		Robitussin-CF	
		Ryna-Tussadine	
		S-T Forte	
		Sinarest	
		Sinubid	
		Sinulin	
		Sinutab	
		Sinutab-II	
		Sinutab with Codeine	
		Triaminic	
		Triaminic DH	
		Triaminic with Codeine	
		Triaminicin	
		Triaminicol	
		Tussagesic	
		Tussaminic	
		Tussanil DH	
		Tuss-Ornade	
		Ursinus Inlay-Tabs	
		Ventaire	
	Protokylol HCl	Actifed-C	
	Pseudoephedrine HCl	Brexin	
		Broncomar	

PSYCHIATRIC SIDE EFFECTS OF MEDICAL DRUGS (Cont.)

General Classification	Generic	Trade Name	Psychiatric Side Effects
Adrenergic (Sympathomimetic) Drugs (Cont.)	Pseudoephedrine HCl (Cont.)	Codimal-L.A.	
		Cotofed	
		CoTylenol	
		D-Feda Gyrocaps	
		Dimacol	
		Emprazil	
		Emprazil-C	
		Fedahist	
		Fedrazil	
		Histalet DM	
		Histalet	
		Histalet X	
		Isoclor	
		Novafed	
		Novafed A	
		Novahistine DMX	
		Nucofed	
		Pseudo-Bid	
		Pseudocot-G Laytabs	
		Pseudo-Hist	
		Rhinosyn	
		Rhinosyn-DM	
		Robitussin-DAC	
		Robitussin-PE	
		Ryna-C	
		Ryna-Cx	
		Sudachlor T.D.	
		Tussend	
Theophylline Derivatives	Aminophylline	Amesec	
		Aminodur Dura-Tabs	
		Mudrane GG	
		Mudrane GG-2	

PSYCHIATRIC SIDE EFFECTS OF MEDICAL DRUGS (Cont.)

General Classification	Generic	Trade Name	Psychiatric Side Effects
Theophylline Derivatives (Cont.)	Aminophylline (Cont.)	Mudrane	
		Mudrane-2	
		Quinamm	
		Somophyllin	
	Dyphylline	Airet	
		Airet L.A.	
		Dilor	
		Dilor-G	
		Emfaseem	
		Lufyllin	
		Lufyllin-EPG	
		Lufyllin-GG	
		Neothylline	
		Neothylline-G	
	Oxtriphylline	Aerolate	
	Theophylline	Bronchobid Duracap	
		Broncomar	
		Bronkodyl	
		Bronkolixir	
		Bronkotabs	
		Bronkotabs-Hafs	
		Dibron	
		Elixicon	
		Elixophyllin	
		Elixophyllin SR	
		Elixophyllin-Kl	
		Fleet Theophyllin	
		Hylate	
		Isofil	
		Isuprel	

PSYCHIATRIC SIDE EFFECTS OF MEDICAL DRUGS (Cont.)

General Classification	Generic	Trade Name	Psychiatric Side Effects
Theophylline Derivatives (Cont.)	Theophylline (Cont.)	Marax	
		Mudrane	
		Quibron	
		Quibron Plus	
		Slo-Phyllin GG	
		Slo-phyllin GG	
		Slo-phyllin Gyrocaps	
		Synophylate	
		Synophylate-GG	
		Synophylate-L.A.	
		Tedral	
		Tedral SA	
		Tedral-25	
		Theobid	
		Theo-Dur	
		Theolair	
		Theo-Organidin	
		Theophyl-225	
		Theospan	
	Theophylline monoethanolamine	Fleet Theophylline	
	Theophylline sodium glycinate	Asbron G Inlay-Tabs	
		Synophylate	
		Synophylate-GG	
Adrenergic-Blocking (Sympatholytic) Drugs	Methysergide maleate	Sansert	Depersonalization
			Depression
			Confusion

PSYCHIATRIC SIDE EFFECTS OF MEDICAL DRUGS (Cont.)

General Classification	Generic	Trade Name	Psychiatric Side Effects
Cholinergic-Blocking (Parasympatholytic) Agents*			General statement regarding cholinergic-blocking agents: agitation nervousness hallucinations disorientation psychosis
			*Symptoms often may be mistaken for senility or mental deterioration caused by progression of the disease in Parkinsonism patients.
	Adiphenine HCl	Transentine Transentine-Phenobarbital	
	Alverine citrate	Spacolin	
	Anisotropine methylbromide	Valpin 50 Valpin 50-PB	
	Atropine sulfate	Antispasmodic Antrocol Arco-Lace Plus Diphenoxylate with atropine Donphen Hybephen Oraminic Spancap Prosed Prydon Trac Tabs Trac Tabs 2x Urised Uristat	Restlessness Irritability Disorientation Incoherence Depression

PSYCHIATRIC SIDE EFFECTS OF MEDICAL DRUGS (Cont.)

General Classification	Generic	Trade Name	Psychiatric Side Effects
Cholinergic-Blocking (Parasympatholytic) Agents (Cont.)			
	Belladonna extract	Belap	
		Oxoids	
		Ro-Bile	
	Belladonna leaf		
	Belladonna leaf fluid extract		
	Belladonna preparations	Barbidonna	
		Belap	
		Belladenal	
		Belladonna Tincture	
		Donnagel	
		Donnagel-PG	
		Donnatal	
		Donnatal Extentabs	
		Donnatal No. 2	
		Donnazyme	
		Donphen	
		Kinesed	
		Prydon Spansule	
		Sidonna	
		Trac Tabs	
		Trac Tabs 2x	
		Uristat	
	Benztropine mesylate	Cogentin	
	Biperiden	Akineton	
	Chlorphenoxamine HCl	Phenoxene HCl	
	Cyrimine HCl	Pagitane HCl	
	Dicyclomine HCl	Bentyl	
		Bentyl with Phenobarbital	
		Dyspas	

PSYCHIATRIC SIDE EFFECTS OF MEDICAL DRUGS (Cont.)

General Classification	Generic	Trade Name	Psychiatric Side Effects
Cholinergic-Blocking (Parasympatholytic) Agents (Cont.)			
	Diphemanil methylsulfate	Prantal	Restlessness
	Ethopropazine HCl	Parsidol HCl	Delirium
			Hallucinations
			Paranoid psychosis
	Glycopyrrolate	Robinul	
		Robinul forte	
		Robinul with Phenobarbital	
		Robinul Forte with Phenobarbital	
	Hexocyclium methylsulfate	Tral Filmtab	
		Tral Gradumet	
	Homatrophine methylbromide	Gustase-Plus	
		Homapin Liquitab	
		Homapin-5	
		Homapin-10	
		Matropinal	
		Metropinal Forte	
		Sed-Tens SE	
		Sinulin	
	Hyoscyamine	Cystospaz	
		Kutrase	
		Levsin	
		Levsin with Phenobarbital	
		Levsinex Timecaps	
		Levsinex with Pehnobarbital	
		Prosed	
		Urised	

PSYCHIATRIC SIDE EFFECTS OF MEDICAL DRUGS (Cont.)

General Classification	Generic	Trade Name	Psychiatric Side Effects
Cholinergic-Blocking (Parasympatholytic) Agents (Cont.)	Hyoscyamine sulfate	Anaspaz	
		Anaspaz PB	
		Antispasmodic Elixir	
		Antispasmodic	
		Arco-Lase Plus	
		Cytospaz-M	
		Cytospaz-SR	
		Donphen	
		Hybephen	
		Hybephen Elixir	
		Levsin	
		Levsin/Phenobarbital Timecaps	
		Prydon Spansule	
		Sidonna	
		Uristat	
	Isometheptene HCl	Octin Hcl	
	Isometheptene mucate	Midrin	
		Octin Mucate	
	Isopropamide iodide	Combid Spansule	
		Darbid	
		Ornade Spansule	
		Tuss-Ornade	
	Mepenzolate bromide	Cantil	
		Cantil with Phenobarbital	
	Methantheline bromide	Bantine Bromide	
	Methixene HCl	Trest	
	Methscopolamine bromide	Hyoscine Methylbromide	
		Pamine Bromide	
		Pamine PB	
		Scopolamine Methylbromide	

PSYCHIATRIC SIDE EFFECTS OF MEDICAL DRUGS (Cont.)

General Classification	Generic	Trade Name	Psychiatric Side Effects
Cholinergic-Blocking (Parasympatholytic) Agents (Cont.)	Methscopolamine nitrate	Extendryl	
		Histaspan-D	
		MSC Triaminic	
		Narine Gyrocaps	
		Paraspan	
		Sinovan Timed	
	Methylatropine nitrate	Atropine Methylnitrate	
		Metropine	
	Orphenadrine citrate	Norflex	
		Norgesic	
		Orforine	
		Orphengesic	
	Orphenadrine HCl	Disipal	
	Oxyphencyclimine HCl	Daricon	
		Daricon PB	
		Enarax	
		Gastrix	
	Oxyphenonium bromide	Antrenyl Bromide	
	Pipenzolate bromide	Piptal	
	Piperidolate HCl	Dactil	
	Poldine methylsulfate	Nacton	
	Procyclidine HCl	Kemadrin	
	Propantheline bromide	Giquel	
		Pro-Banthine	
		Pro-Banthine PA	
		Pro-Banthine with Dartal	
		Probanthine with Phenobarbital	
		Propantheline Bromide with Phenobarbital	

PSYCHIATRIC SIDE EFFECTS OF MEDICAL DRUGS (Cont.)

General Classification	Generic	Trade Name	Psychiatric Side Effects
Cholinergic-Blocking (Parasympatholytic) Agents (Cont.)	Scopolamine hydrobromide	Donphen Hyoscine Hydrobromide Prydon Scopolamine Hydrobromide Sidonna	Disorientation Delirium
	Thiphenamil HCl Tridihexethyl chloride	Trocinate Milpath Pathibamate Pathilon	
	Trihexyphenidyl HCl	Antitrem Artane Artane Sequels Hexyphen 5 Pipanol Tremin	Psychosis
Mydriatics and Cycloplegics	Atropine sulfate	Atropisol BufOpto Atropine Isopto Atropine	General statement regarding mydriatics and cycloplegics: irritability
	Cyclopentolate HCl Homatropine hydrobromide	Cyclogyl BufOpto Homatrocel Isopto Homatropine	hyperactivity confusion hallucinations
	Scopolamine Tropicamide	Isopto Hyoscine Mydriacyl	delirium

PSYCHIATRIC SIDE EFFECTS OF MEDICAL DRUGS (Cont.)

General Classification	Generic	Trade Name	Psychiatric Side Effects
Insulin and Oral Antidiabetics			
Insulins	Extended insulin zinc suspension	Ultralente Iletin Ultralente Insulin	General statement regarding insulins:
			nervousness
	Globin zinc insulin injection		confusion
	Insulin injection	Crystalline Zinc Insulin Regular Iletin Regular Insulin	diminished coordination psychosis
	Insulin zinc suspension	Iletin, Lente Iletin, Semilente Iletin, Ultralente Insulin, Lente Insulin, Protamine Zinc Insulin, Semilente Insulin, Ultralente Protamine, Zinc, & Iletin	
	Isophane insulin suspension	NPH Iletin NPH Insulin	
Oral Antidiabetic Agents	Acetohexamide Chlorpropamide Phenformin HCl	Dymelor Diabinese DBI DBI-TD Meltrol	General statement regarding oral antidiabetic agents: confusion paresthesia
	Tolazamide Tolbutamide	Tolinase Ornase	

PSYCHIATRIC SIDE EFFECTS OF MEDICAL DRUGS (Cont.)

General Classification	Generic	Trade Name	Psychiatric Side Effects
Thyroid and Antithyroid Drugs			
Thyroid Preparations	Levothyroxine sodium	Cytolen Letter Levoid Ro-Thyroxin Synthroid I-Thyroxine Sodium	General statement regarding thyroid preparations: nervousness agitation hyperirritability insomnia twitching tremor
	Liothyronine sodium	Cytomel Ro-thyronine Sodium-I-Triiodothyronine	
	Thyroglobulin	Proloid	
	Thyroid	Armour Thyroid Euthroid Thyrolar	
	Thyroid desiccated	Dried Thyroid S-P-T Thyrar Thyrocrine Thyroglandular Thyroid Extract ThyroTeric	
	Thyrotropin	Thytropar	
Adrenocorticosteroids and Analogs*	Betamethasone Betamethasone benzoate	Celestone Benisone Flurobate Uticort	General statement regarding adrenocorticosteroids and analogs: euphoria manic-depressive states psychosis
	Betamethasone valerate Corticotropin	Valisone ACTH Acthar	*Aggravation of existing emotional instability or psychotic tendencies

PSYCHIATRIC SIDE EFFECTS OF MEDICAL DRUGS (Cont.)

General Classification	Generic	Trade Name	Psychiatric Side Effects
Adrenocorticosteroids and Analogs (Cont.)	Corticotropin (Cont.)	Adrenocorticotropic Hormone Cortigel Cortrophin Compound E Cortone Acetate	
	Cortisone acetate		
	Desoxycorticosterone acetate	DOCA Acetate Percorten Percorten Pellets	
	Desoxycorticosterone pivalate	Percorten Pivalate	
	Dexamethasone	Aeroseb-Dex Decaderm in Estergel Decadron Deronil Dexone Gammacorten Hexodrol SK-Dexamethasone	
	Dexamethasone acetate	Decadron-La Delladec	
	Dexamethasone sodium phosphate	Decadron Phosphate Deksone Delladec Dexasone Dezone Hexadrol Phosphate	

PSYCHIATRIC SIDE EFFECTS OF MEDICAL DRUGS (Cont.)

General Classification	Generic	Trade Name	Psychiatric Side Effects
Adrenocorticosteroids and Analogs (Cont.)			
	Fludrocortisone acetate	Florinef	
	Flumethasone pivalate	Locorten	
	Flucinolone acetonide	Fluonid	
		Neo-Synalar	
		Synalar	
		Synalar-HP	
		Synemol	
	Fluocinonide	Lidex	
		Lidex-E	
		Topsyn	
	Fluorometholone	Neo-Oxylone	
		Oxylone	
	Fluprednisolone	Alphadrol	
	Hydrocortisone	Aeroseb-HC	
		Allersone	
		Alphosyl-HC	
		Biocort Otic	
		Carmol HC	
		Cort-Dome	
		Cortef	
		Cortenema	
		Corticaine	
		Cortisporin	
		Cortril	
		Cotacort	
		Dek-Quin	
		Dermacort	
		Formtone-HC	
		Hydrocortisone	
		Hytone	
		Loroxide-HC	

PSYCHIATRIC SIDE EFFECTS OF MEDICAL DRUGS (Cont.)

General Classification	Generic	Trade Name	Psychiatric Side Effects
Adrenocorticosteroids and Analogs (Cont.)	Hydrocortisone (Cont.)	Orlex HC	
		Otic Neo-Cort-Dome	
		Otobione	
		Otocort	
		Proctocort	
		Pyocidin-Otic	
		Racet	
		Racet LCD	
		Rectoid	
		Terra-Cortril Spray with Polymyxin B Sulfate	
		Texacort Scalp Lotion	
		Vanoxide-HC	
		Vioform-Hydrocortisone	
		Vosol HC Otic	
		Vytone	
		Ze-Tar-Quin	
		Zetone	
	Hydrocortisone acetate	Anusol-HC	
		Carmol HC	
		Coly-Mycin S Otic with Neomycin and Hydro-cortisone	
		Cort-Dome	
		Cortef Acetate Ointment	
		Cortisporin	
		Derma Medicone-HC	
		Komed HC	
		Mantadil	
		Neo-Cortef	
		Orabase HCA	

PSYCHIATRIC SIDE EFFECTS OF MEDICAL DRUGS (Cont.)

General Classification	Generic	Trade Name	Psychiatric Side Effects
Adrenocorticosteroids and Analogs (Cont.)			
	Hydrocortisone acetate (Cont.)	Pramosone	
		Protofoam-HC	
		Rectal Medicone-HC	
		Terra-Cortril	
		Cortef Fluid	
	Hydrocortisone cypionate		
	Hydrocortisone sodium phosphate	Hydrocortone Phosphate	
	Hydrocortisone sodium succinate	A-hydro Cort	
		Solu-Cortef	
	Hydrocortamate HCl	Ulcort	
	Methylprednisolone	Medrol	
		Neo-Medrol	
	Methylprednisolone acetate	Depo-Medrol	
		Medrol Acetate	
		Medrol Enpak	
		Neo-Medrol Acetate	
	Methylprednisolone sodium succinate	A-MethaPred	
		Solu-Medrol	
	Paramethasone acetate	Haldrone	
		Stemex	
		Stero-Darvon with ASA	
	Prednisolone	Delta-Cortef	
		Meticortelone	
		Meti-Derm	
		Prednisolone	
		Sterale	
		Sterane	

PSYCHIATRIC SIDE EFFECTS OF MEDICAL DRUGS (Cont.)

General Classification	Generic	Trade Name	Psychiatric Side Effects
Adrenocorticosteroids and Analogs (Cont.)			
	Prednisolone acetate	Meticortelone Acetate	
		Metimyd	
		Neo-Delta-Cortef	
		Nisolone	
		Savacort	
		Sterane	
	Prednisolone sodium phosphate	Hydeltrasol	
		Metreton	
		Optimyd	
		PSP-IV	
		Savacort-S	
		Sodasone	
	Prednisolone sodium succinate	Meticortelone Soluble	
	Prednisolone tebutate	Hydeltra-TBA	
	Prednisone	Delta-Dome	
		Deltasone	
		Meticorten	
		Paracort	
		Prednisone	
		Servisone	
		SK-Prednisone	
		Sterapred Uni-Pak	
	Triamcinolone	Aristocort	
		Kenacort	
		Rocinolone	
	Triamcinolone acetonide	Aristocort A	
		Aristoderm	
		Kenalog	
		Mycolog	
	Triamcinolone diacetate	Aristocort Diacetate	
		Cenocort Forte	

PSYCHIATRIC SIDE EFFECTS OF MEDICAL DRUGS (Cont.)

General Classification	Generic	Trade Name	Psychiatric Side Effects
Adrenocorticosteroids and Analogs (Cont.)	Triamcinolone diacetate (Cont.)	Cino-40 Kenacort Aristospan	General statement regarding estrogens:
	Triamcinolone hexacetonide		irritabiltiy
			depression
			paresthesia
Estrogens, Progestins and Oral Contraceptives			lassitude
Estrogens	Benzestrol	Chemestrogen	anxiety
	Chlorotrianisene	Tace	insomnia
	Dienestrol	AVC/Dienestrol	
	Diethylstilbestrol	DES	
		Stilbestrol	
		Tylosterone	
	Diethylstilbestrol diphosphate	Stilphostrol	
	Diethylstilbestrol diproprionate		
	Estradiol	Aquadiol	
		Estrace	
		Progynon Pellets	
		Test-Estrin	
	Estradiol benzoate		
	Estradiol cypionate	Depa-Estradiol Cypionate	
		E-Ionate	
		Femogen	
	Estradiol dipropionate	Delestrogen	
	Estradiol valerate	Ditate-DS	
		Duratrad	
		Estate	
		Estraval PA	
		Femogen LA	
		Rep-Estra	

PSYCHIATRIC SIDE EFFECTS OF MEDICAL DRUGS (Cont.)

General Classification	Generic	Trade Name	Psychiatric Side Effects
Estrogens (Cont.)	Estrogens conjugated	Milprem	
		Premarin	
	Esterified estrogens	Amnestrogen	
		Estratab	
		Evex	
		Femogen	
		Menest	
		Menrium	
		SK-Estrogens	
	Estrone	Estrusol	
		Menformin (A)	
		Theelin	
		Wynestron	
	Estrone piperazine sulfate	Ogen	
	Estrone potassium sulfate	Fernspan	
		Spanestrin P	
		Theelin R-P	
	Ethinyl estradiol	Brevicon	
		Demulen	
		Estinyl	
		Feminone	
		Gevrine	
		Gynetone	
		Loestrin	
		Lo/Ovral	
		Lynoral	
		Modicon	
		Nolestrin	
		Os-Cal Mone	
		Ovcon	
		Ovral	

PSYCHIATRIC SIDE EFFECTS OF MEDICAL DRUGS (Cont.)

General Classification	Generic	Trade Name	Psychiatric Side Effects
Estrogens (Cont.)	Ethinyl estradiol (Cont.)	Testand-B Zorane	
		Vallestril	
	Hexestrol	Estradurin	
	Methallenestril	Meprane Dipropionate	
	Polyestradiol phosphate		
	Promethestrol dipropionate		
Estrogen-Progestin Combinations (Oral Contraceptives)		Brevicon Demulen Envoid Loestrin Lo/Ovral Modicon Norinyl Norlestrin Ortho-Novum Ovulen Ovral Zorane	General statement regarding estrogen-progestin combinations: marked mood swings
Progestin Only (Contraceptives)		Micronor Nor QD Ovrette	

PSYCHIATRIC SIDE EFFECTS OF MEDICAL DRUGS (Cont.)

General Classification	Generic	Trade Name	Psychiatric Side Effects
Diuretics			
Carbonic Anhydrase Inhibitor Diuretics	Acetazolamide	Diamox	General statement regarding carbonic anhydrase inhibitor diuretics:
		Hydrazol	irritability
		Daranid	disorientation
	Dichlorphenamide	Oratrol	
		Cardrase	
	Ethoxzolamide	Ethamide	
		Neptazane	
	Methazolamide		
Xanthines	Theobromine calcium salicylate	Theocalcin	General statement regarding Xanthines:
	Theobromine magnesium oleate	Athemol	nervousness
		Athemol-N	insomnia
			restlessness
			irritability
			delirium
Miscellaneous Agents	Ethacrynic acid	Edecrin	Confusion
	Spironolactone	Aldactazide	Apprehension
		Aldactone	Confusion
Histamine/Antihistamines			
Antihistamines	Bromodiphenhydramine	Ambodryl	General statement regarding antihistamines:
	Brompheniramine maleate	Brocon C.R.	decreased coordination
		Dimetane	paradoxical excitation—
		Dimetane-Ten	expecially in children:
		Dimetapp	restlessness
		Dimetapp Extentabs	insomnia
		Histatapp	tremor
		Histatapp T.D.	

PSYCHIATRIC SIDE EFFECTS OF MEDICAL DRUGS (Cont.)

General Classification	Generic	Trade Name	Psychiatric Side Effects
Antihistamines (Cont.)	Brompheniramine maleate (Cont.)	Puretane	euphoria
		Puretapp	nervousness
		Puretapp-PA	delirium
	Carbinoxamine maleate	Clistin	epileptiform seizures
		Rondec	personality changes
		Rondec-DM	hallucinations
	Chlorpheniramine maleate	Alka-Seltzer Plus	
		Allerest	
		Chlor-Trimeton	
		Chlor-Trimeton with Codeine	
		Chlor-Trimeton Repetabs	
		Codimal L.A.	
		Colrex	
		Coricidin	
		Coricidin D	
		Coriforte	
		Corilin	
		CoTylenol	
		Deconamine	
		Decongest T.D.	
		Demazin Repetabs	
		Extendryl	
		Fedahist	
		Guistrey Fortis	
		Histabid Duracap	
		Histalet DM	
		Histalet Forte	
		Histaspan	
		Histaspan-D	
		Histaspan-Plus	
		Isoclor	

PSYCHIATRIC SIDE EFFECTS OF MEDICAL DRUGS (Cont.)

General Classification	Generic	Trade Name	Psychiatric Side Effects
Antihistamines (Cont.)	Chlorpheniramine maleate (Cont.)	Korigesic	
		Kronohist Kronocaps	
		Matropinal	
		Naldecon	
		Napril Plateau Caps	
		Narine Gyrocaps	
		Neotep Granucaps	
		Nolamine	
		Novafed	
		Novahistine	
		Oraminic	
		Ornade	
		Pediacof	
		Pseudo-Hist	
		Quelidrine	
		Rhinex D-Lay	
		Rhinex	
		Rhinex DM	
		Rhinosyn	
		Rhinosyn-DM	
		Ryna-C	
		Ryna-Tussadine	
		Sinarest	
		Singlet	
		Sinovan Timed	
		Sinulin	
		Sudachlor T.D.	
		Teldrin	
		Triaminicin	
		Tusquelin	

General Classification	Generic	Trade Name	Psychiatric Side Effects
Antihistamines (Cont.)	Chlorpheniramine maleate (Cont.)	Tussanil DH	
		Tussi-Organidin	
		Tussi-Organidin DM	
		Tuss-Ornade	
	Cyclizine HCl	Marezine Hydrochloride	
		Migral	
	Cyclizine lactate	Marezine Lactate	
	Cyproheptadine HCL	Periactin	
	Dexbrompheniramine maleate	Disomer	
		Disophrol Chronotab	
		Drixoral	
	Dexchlorpheniramine maleate	Polaramine	
	Dimenhydrinate	Dimenest	
		Dramamine	
		Meni-D	
		Reidamine	
	Dimethindene maleate	Forhistal Maleate	
		Triten	
	Diphenhydramine HCl	Bax	
		Benadryl	
		Benylin	
		Diphenadril	
		Fenylhist	
		Rohydra	
		SK-Diphenhydramine	
		Valdrene	
	Diphenylpyraline HCl	Diafen	
		Hispril	
	Doxylamine succinate	Bendectin	
		Decapryn	

PSYCHIATRIC SIDE EFFECTS OF MEDICAL DRUGS (Cont.)

General Classification	Generic	Trade Name	Psychiatric Side Effects
Antihistamines (Cont.)	Meclizine HCl	Antivert	
		Bonine	
		Meclizine	
	Methapyrilene HCl	Brexin	
		Citra	
		Citra Forte	
		Co-Pyronil	
		Ephed-Organidin	
		Hista-Clopane	
		Histadyl	
		Histadyl Pulvules	
	Methdilazine HCl	Tacaryl HCl	
	Promethazine HCl	Lemprometh	
		Phenergan	
		Phenergan with Codeine	
		Phenergan with Dextro-methorphan	
		Phenergan VC	
		Phenergan VC with Codeine	
		Promethazine with Codeine	
		Quadnite	
		Remsed	
		Synalgos	
		Synalgos-DC	
		ZiPan	
	Pyrilamine maleate	Allerest	
		Citra	
		Citra Forte	
		Codimal DH	
		Codimal DM	
		Codimal PH	

PSYCHIATRIC SIDE EFFECTS OF MEDICAL DRUGS (Cont.)

General Classification	Generic	Trade Name	Psychiatric Side Effects
Antihistamines (Cont.)	Pyrilamine maleate (Cont.)	Eme-Nil	
		Emesert	
		4-Way Nasal Spray	
		Fiogesic	
		Histalet Forte	
		Kronohist Kronocaps	
		MSC Triaminic	
		Matropinal	
		Matropinal Forte	
		Napril Plateau Caps	
		Ryna-Tussadine	
		Sunril	
		Triaminic	
		Triaminic DH	
		Triaminic with Codeine	
		Tussagesic	
		Tussaminic	
		Tussanil DH	
		Ursinus	
		Wans	
	Trimeprazine tartrate	Temaril	
	Tripelennamine citrate	Pyribenzamine Citrate	
	Tripelennamine HCl	PBZ-SR	
		Pyribenzamine Hcl	
		Rhulihist	
	Triprolidine HCl	Actidil	
		Actifed-C	

PSYCHIATRIC SIDE EFFECTS OF MEDICAL DRUGS (Cont.)

General Classification	Generic	Trade Name	Psychiatric Side Effects
Vitamins			
Vitamin B Complex	Leucovorin	Calcium Leucovorin Folinic Acid	Diminished concentration Altered sleep patterns Irritability Hyperactivity Excitement Depression Confusion Impaired judgment
Antitussives and Expectorants			
Nonnarcotic antitussives	Chlophedianol HCl	Ulo	Excitation Hyperirritability Nightmares Hallucinations
Expectorants	Ammonium chloride	Benylin Coricidin Diphenadril Quelidrine Rhinex DM Triaminicol Zypan	Confusion Excitement Hyperventilation
Antidiarrheal Agents			
Systemic Agents	Diphenoxylate	Lomotil	Euphoria Depression

PSYCHIATRIC SIDE EFFECTS OF MEDICAL DRUGS (Cont.)

General Classification	Generic	Trade Name	Psychiatric Side Effects
Emetics/Antiemetics			
Antiemetics	Diphenidol hcl	Vontrol	Hallucinations
			Disorientation
			Confusion
Miscellaneous Agents	Carbidopa/levodopa	Sinemet	Twisting of tongue
			Grimacing
			Waving of hands, neck and feet
			Bruxism
			Jerky and involuntary movements
			Dyskinesia
			Agitation
			Anxiety
			Confusion
			Depression
			Antisocial behavior
			Suicidal tendencies
			Increased libido
			Mood swings
	Levodopa	Bendopa	Grimacing
		Bio/Dopa	Bruxism
		Dopar	Twisting of tongue
		Larodopa	Waving of neck, hands and feet
		L-dopa	Jerky and involuntary movements

TABLE 1. PSYCHIATRIC SIDE EFFECTS OF MEDICAL DRUGS (Cont.)

General Classification	Generic	Trade Name	Psychiatric Side Effects
Miscellaneous Agents (Cont.)	Levodopa (Cont.)	Sinemet	Dyskinesia
			Agitation
			Anxiety
			Confusion
			Depression
			Antisocial behavior
			Suicidal tendencies
			Increased libido
			Mood swings

Index